CW01316745

THE SLIM FACTOR

Julie Dargan RN, ND, BHSc

authorHOUSE®

AuthorHouse™ UK Ltd.
500 Avebury Boulevard
Central Milton Keynes, MK9 2BE
www.authorhouse.co.uk
Phone: 08001974150

© 2011. Julie Dargan. All rights reserved

No part of this book may be reproduced, stored in a retrieval system, or transmitted by any means without the written permission of the author.

First published by AuthorHouse   02/18/2011

ISBN: 978-1-4567-7416-5 (sc)
ISBN: 978-1-4567-7417-2 (hc)

Any people depicted in stock imagery provided by Thinkstock are models, and such images are being used for illustrative purposes only. Certain stock imagery © Thinkstock.

This book is printed on acid-free paper.

Because of the dynamic nature of the Internet, any Web addresses or links contained in this book may have changed since publication and may no longer be valid. The views expressed in this work are solely those of the author and do not necessarily reflect the views of the publisher, and the publisher hereby disclaims any responsibility for them.

To Jim, Banjo and Jake

My life is not measured by the number of breaths I have taken, but by the number of people who took my breath away. This book is dedicated to those people.

Contents

Preface	xi
Introducing the slim factor concept	1
What the slim factor program will do for you.	3
Set point theory	4
Why some people are overweight, yet eat very little, while others can eat anything they like and still not put on weight?	7
Testimonies	8

PART ONE

CHAPTER 1

Introducing leptin: the messenger between the hypothalamus and the fat stores.	11
Leptin some simple facts	12
What happens when leptin levels fall?	14
Summary of chapter one	15

CHAPTER TWO

Leptin resistance: a weight loss nightmare	17
Summary of chapter two	21

CHAPTER 3

Why are people leptin resistant?	23

1. High fructose corn syrup.
2. C-reactive Protein.
3. Hydrogenated fats.
4. Mono-sodium glutamate.
5. Aspartamine.
6. Carbohydrate foods.
7. Other sugar substitutes.
8. Other reasons.

Why does the body allow leptin resistance to occur?	30
Summary of chapter three.	32

CHAPTER FOUR

The diencephalon introducing Dr. A.T.W. Simeons	33
The hypothalamus	34
The Slim Factor in action	36
Aim of Slim Factor program	38
Summary of chapter four	39

CHAPTER FIVE

Abnormal fats vs normal fats	41
Thyroid myths	43
Summary of chapter five	44

CHAPTER SIX

What is hCG?	45
Homeopathic hCG.	47
Summary of chapter six	48

CHAPTER SEVEN

Objectives of the Slim Factor Program	49
The Slim Factor Program.	51
How does the Slim Factor Program work?	53
Very low calorie diet vs very low calorie diet with hcg.	54
Summary of chapter seven	55

CHAPTER EIGHT

Starting the program: Simple tasks before you start the program	57
Summary of one cycle of the Program	59

PART TWO

CHAPTER NINE

The Program: Phase 1, Step 1: Loading Phase	63
How to take the drops	65
Phase 1, Step 2: VLCD	66
Sample diet day.	69
Activities to incorporate into the program	70
What to expect on the program?	73
How to overcome any stalling in weight loss.	75

CHAPTER TEN

Frequently asked questions   77
1. Will I be hungry on this program?
2. I am suffering from constipation, what can I do?
3. Why do I have muscle fatigue?
4. Why am I suffering from headaches?
5. Will I suffer with sagging skin once the weight is lost?
6. Some diet protocols promote the use of Stevia. Why is this not included in The Slim Factor program?
7. Can I do the program if I am pregnant?
8. Why am I experiencing leg cramps?
9. If hCG is released during pregnancy, why are pregnant women not losing weight during their pregnancy?
10. What do I do if I want to lose more weight?

CHAPTER ELEVEN

Phase 2: Maintenance Phase	83
Resetting your Set Point	84
Foods to avoid while on the Maintenance Phase	86
What you are allowed to eat while on three week maintenance phase.	87

PART THREE

CHAPTER TWELVE
Program for the rest of your life   93
Tips for a healthy digestion.   96

CHAPTER THIRTEEN
Are you getting enough exercise?   99
Benefits of walking.   101
Techniques to remember while walking   102
Reasons for walking   103

CHAPTER FOURTEEN
Specific reasons <u>not</u> do this program   105

CHAPTER FIFTEEN
Recipes while on the VLCD.   107
Soups/juices   108
Lunch/dinners   110
Desserts   114
Recipes while on the Maintenace Phase   115

PART FOUR

APPENDIX ONE
1. Daily allowance   119
2. Caloric count   121
3. Supplements   123
   - Coconut oil
   - Raw Apple Cider Vinegar
   - Pro-biotics
   - Green Tea
   - Nopal Cactus
   - Spirulina, Wheatgrass & Chlorella
   - Vitamin & Mineral Complex
   - Cinnamon
   - Essential Fatty Acids
   - Magnesium

- Yerba Mate Tea
- Pu-Erh Tea

4. The Slim Factor personal weight loss tracking chart.   131
5. The Slim Factor Personal Measurement tracking chart.   133
6. The Slim Factor Personal body mass index (BMI) calculator   135
7. Conversions   137
8. Monosodium glutamate (MSG)   139
9. High fructose corn syrup (HFCS)   145

Glossary   147
Resources   153
Bibliography   155

List of Tables

1. Benefits of this nutritional program.   3
2. Leptin's major regulatory roles.   13
3. Symptoms of leptin resistance   18
4. Complications due to increased leptin levels.   31
5. Causes of Hypothalamic Impairment   35
6. Lipogenesis vs lipolysis   48
7. Diseases that improve while taking hCG   48
8. How to overcome stalling   75
9. One cycle of The Slim Factor Program   85

List of Illustrations

1. Flow Sheet of Leptin resistance.   32
2. Sample diet day.   119

PREFACE

This is my remarkable story and one that I hope will inspire everyone who reads this book. It is the story of my journey but you can make it your journey too. In this book you will have a world of resources at your fingertips in order for you to become the person you want to be, not the person that people have decided who you are to be.

Let me share with you some of my background. I am a wife and mother with a wonderful husband and two beautiful boys. I was a Registered Nurse for 20 years before embarking on a career in preventative medicine. So, after the birth of my second child at the age of 38, it was back to the school books for me where I studied Naturopathy for another six years. At the final end of all my studies I am now a Naturopath (encompassing Nutrition and Herbs with Homeopathy and Massage) with a Bachelor of Health Sciences under my belt. The relief at the end of the studies was enormous but with it came the realisation of how much weight I had gained.

This weight gain had me baffled. After years of studying Naturopathy I had the best diet ever, yet I was tipping into the obesity level of Body Mass Index (BMI), which had me very worried. What was I doing wrong? I was approaching 45 years of age and knew that if I did not get a grip of my ever expanding waistline, once menopause kicked in, I would really be in trouble.

Now I am not one for diets. I always, and still do, believe that if weight has to be lost it has to mean a change in how one interacts with their food, as well as incorporating a good exercise program. I had a good look at my diet, cut out on all snacks, upped the exercise, drank plenty of water, stopped the alcohol and guess what?? Nothing happened. No weight loss, no feeling good about myself, nothing. I kept this up for a couple of months only to get despondent. Why put myself through all this torture and self restraint if I was going to have nothing to show for it?

I remember saying to my husband that this is it. "This is how I am going to be and so you had better get used to it. Some people are meant to be skinny while others simply over the years pile on the pounds so slowly and so insidiously that nothing can be done about it. It is all a part of the ageing process." Not the right attitude I admit but I was willing to admit defeat at this stage. Then came the Tipping Point, the point I knew I could no longer ignore my expanding waistline.

I can still remember the turning point for me. It was May 2010 and we were having a summer party. There was nothing decent in the wardrobe that I could wear as I had slowly been putting on the weight and would wear elastic waist trousers all the time. I decided to buy myself a nice summer dress as the weather was proving to be warm on the day in question. Well, and this is still very emotional for me to admit, there was nothing in any of the shops that would fit me. For the first time I came to the realisation that I was now considered obese, and therefore all my usual clothes shops did not have anything in my size.

What I had not realised was that while I was focusing on how big my tummy was getting with my ever expanding waistline, I had not realised there were other areas of my body where fat was accumulating. This would include shoulders, thighs, hips, face, you name the area and the fat was getting deposited there. Dresses would not go over my shoulders. In some change rooms, I had trouble getting the dress off once I had stupidly insisted would look great on me if I could simply get it over my shoulders. I was getting hot and flustered and, regrettably, had to admit defeat in finding an outfit for the day. I was no longer in denial; reality had hit me hard and fast.

It would have been a week later when I came across an article by a Dr. A. T. W. Simeons, *Pounds & Inches: A new approach to obesity*. He was a British endocrinologist and dedicated 40 years of his life seeking the underlying cause to obesity. The article was written in the 1950's and much of what he wrote at the time about how his diet worked was not understood. This book will unite the old with the new to give you a better idea as to what is going on in YOUR body.

Before I started this program I was reaching size 18 and tipping into the obesity section of the BMI chart with a BMI of 30.5 Five months later I was a size 10 with a BMI of 22 putting me into a normal range. Yippee, all that hard work and perseverance finally paid off. I looked great, I felt great. People commented on how great I looked. My skin tone was rejuvenated; there was a fresh sparkle in my eyes. One day I realised it was not the weight loss that people were focusing on but on how great I looked. Those words only made my confidence soar higher. I had not anticipated how great I would feel, how much energy I would have, and it felt good. It felt great to be alive. Not only had I lost the weight, but it has also stayed off.

Before anyone wants to begin a program you want to make sure that the program has been properly vetted and validated with appropriate double-blind studies. Dr Daniel Belluscio, MD, Director of The Oral hCG research Centre in Argentina has successfully demonstrated consistent results with hCG. Records in his clinics show well over 6,000 patients. The program I am going to share with you has been proven to be an effective method for obesity management by being validated by appropriate double-blind studies.

- D. Belluscio, et al, *Utility of an Oral presentation of hCG for the Management of Obesity. A double-blind study.* The Oral hCG Research Clinic. Accessed 14 November 2010. http://hcgobesity.org/research/index.html.
- W. L. Asher, Harold W. Harper, Effect of human chorionic gonadotrophin on weight loss, hunger, and feeling of well-being. *American Journal of Clinical Nutrition*, (26); 211-18, Accessed 14 November, 2010. http://www.ajcn.org/cgi/content/abstract/26/2/211

My sons are very open about how great their Mummy now looks. They told me how much better I was to hug as they now could now get their arms around me when they hugged me. Funny the honest comments children make. I am more relaxed with my children; I have more energy to do things with them. The dog is enjoying the big walks I am now able to undertake. The minor aches that were starting to creep in that we all put down to the ageing process, are now gone.

The diet industry is forever booming with over $20 billion being spent annually on diets and diet products in America alone. This industry would collapse if it became widely known that obesity is a **permanently curable symptom** of a hypothalamus dysfunction. This book is going to explain just why people are obese and how to overcome any hypothalamic dysfunction.

On a final note, Leonardo Da Vinci was once asked how he creates such wonders as the Statue of David that proudly stands on display in Florence. His response was that he just chips away at the marble and the figure emerges. The figure was always there, waiting to be revealed. That is exactly how I feel. I needed something to chip away at the fat padding that was encasing my body, to reveal the new me. In this book I will share with you my secret to help you to reveal the NEW YOU!

INTRODUCING THE SLIM FACTOR CONCEPT

There is no denying in the fact that we as a population are getting bigger as each year goes by.

The following statistics are taken from the World Health Organisation's website. (Accessed November 14th 2010.)

WHO's latest projections indicate that globally in 2005:
- Approximately 1.6 billion adults (age 15+) were overweight;
- At least 400 million adults were obese.
- WHO further projects that by 2015, approximately 2.3 billion adults will be overweight and more than 700 million will be obese.
- At least 20 million children under the age of five years are overweight globally in 2005.

Experts all have their own opinion on what are the major causes of why obesity is becoming such a problem. One does not have to be a rocket scientist to work out just why we are getting bigger. All you have to do is look at the sizes of portions of meals we are now eating. If you are a fast food eater you may be surprised by the following changes in meal sizes:

- In the 1950's a Burger King burger was 2.8oz and 202 calories, in 2004 it is 4.9oz and 400 calories.
- McDonald's fry's were 2.4 oz and 210 calories, now 7oz and 455 calories.
- Anyone remember the Coco-Cola bottles from 1916? Just 6.5 fl.oz and 70 calories, now the smallest bottle available is 16 fl oz and 194 calories. A can of Coco-cola is 240mls with 140 calories.
- Popcorn at the movies? In the 1950's they were 3 cups and 174 calories. Now they are a whopping 21 cups and 1,200 calories laden with fats and chemicals!! Who really needs 21 cups of popcorn?

The above foods may be obvious as to why we may be putting on weight but what about people who do not fall into the junk food trap? All you have to do is look at our food pyramids and see that there is an overemphasis on grains/carbohydrates. Then to add insult to injury we are being bombarded with advertisement slogans stating that honey enriched, chocolate coated cereals are full of whole grains allowing us to be deluded into the fact that we are eating healthy. Western diets promote an increase in the consumption of refined foods, high carbohydrates, high sugars, high adulterated fats, alongside nutrient depleted foods. Mix this with physical inactivity and the results are disastrous for our health.

We are celebrating an increase in technology such as washing machines and elevators thus creating a decrease in physical exertion. Very few people walk to work, to school, to the local shops or even to the clothesline! Increased prosperity leads to an increase in calorie consumption, as well as an intensive marketing of sweets, biscuits and fast foods. No wonder we are getting bigger. In fact, how is it possible that anyone is thin in this day and age?

Our expanding waistlines, along with the rest of our bodies, threaten the healthcare systems and puts excessive financial pressure on country's economies. Overweight and obesity lead to serious health consequences. Health risks increase progressively as BMI increases. Raised body mass index is a major risk factor for chronic diseases such as:

- Cardiovascular disease (mainly heart disease and stroke) - already the world's number one cause of death, killing 17 million people each year.
- Diabetes –WHO projects deaths due to diabetic complications will increase by more than 50% worldwide in the next ten years.
- Musculoskeletal disorders – especially osteoarthritis.
- Some cancers (endometrial, breast, and colon).
- Stroke
- Liver disease

WHAT THE SLIM FACTOR PROGRAM WILL DO FOR YOU.

Table One: Benefits of The Slim Factor Program

BENEFITS OF THE NUTRITIONAL PROGRAM
• Weight loss guaranteed. • Lose abnormal fat deposits. • Body is reshaped. Targets the flabby areas on the belly, buttocks, thighs, underarms and chest. Targets the unwanted back fat near the bra line. • No unwanted loss of muscle and structural fat. • Improves muscle tone. • Look and feel great. • Tightens and firms skin, reducing the appearance of cellulite. • Decreases the cravings for carbohydrates and sugar. • Can increase libido in men and women. • Strengthens brittle nails. • Decrease cholesterol levels. • Reduce pain associated with arthritis. • Joint and knee aches disappear. • Blood pressure levels move into a healthy range. • Blood sugar levels, triglycerides and cholesterol levels normalise. • Improvement in sleep patterns. • Skin tone rejuvenated. • Do not gain weight back again once the 23 day program is correctly implemented and 21 day maintenance is adhered to. • Men lose an average 30lb in 23 days. • Women lose an average 25lbs in 23 days. • Requires no specific exercise routine. • No specific dietary formulas. • Feel more comfortable in yourself and wear the clothes you want to wear.

SET POINT THEORY

The Slim Factor program will reset your hypothalamus gland, the gland which regulates the storage of body fat as well as nurturing other glands such as the thyroid and adrenals. Don't think of this program as just a diet. This program helps reset your metabolism and your fat regulation system so your body no longer stores unneeded fat. You will be resetting your metabolism into one of fat burning mode rather than one of fat storage mode.

Once you have completed the program and dropped in both pounds and inches, the hypothalamus will reset your body's set point. This is very important. Research has shown that the human body may have a genetically determined set-point weight that is controlled by metabolic hormones and fat cell enzymes. What this basically means is that after the onset of adulthood the body will maintain a constant level of body fat. This involves a complex set of interactions between the brain, nervous system and the fat cells. This communication can cause a reduction in metabolism when the fat cells signal that too much fat has been lost, for example during a period of dieting and/or exercising. Following a weight loss diet for a period of time will trigger the body to cling to its set point making you put back on the weight plus a little more in case you try this on the body again!

After most diet programs, the body's metabolism can decrease. Your set point is not in control of your destiny. With this program you can reset your body's set point and be in control of your destiny.

In conclusion, there is a strong body of evidence that suggests that each individual has a predetermined weight set point.(e.g. your weight being 180lb). Your individual set point may be difficult to overcome. In this example, you were 180lb and then lost 20lb on a diet. The body will try and put back on the 20lb you lost in order to reach its set point once you finished the diet. However, the majority of people who followed this program and not give up eventually press past their set point closer to their desired weight, which may be 145lb and not putting any weight back on once The Slim Factor program is completed. The actions you take and the level of persistence you demonstrate will determine whether you can conquer your set point.

The Slim Factor program, in combination with products recommended, causes your body to release its stored fat cells, but not all fat cells, just the abnormal fat cells. The abnormal fat cells are the ones you do not need or want. There will be no loss of any vital structural fat or muscle. Not only will you notice a loss in weight but also will notice inches will be lost from the body. Shoulders will appear, rolls from the back will disappear, and hips will be noticeably smaller. The Slim Factor program creates a new mind set within you and can help you reset your satiety centre in the body and get your metabolism burning the extra pounds away. This is a program not just for quick weight loss but a **life style change that will be permanent and lasting**.

Set point theory:

The point at which the body maintains a certain weight by means of its own internal controls.

This book will explain to you why diets in the past did not work, or were short lived. That is, the weight simply was regained once the diet was stopped. One reason being due to the fact that the set point was never adjusted. Statistics have shown that the answer to weight loss does not always work with diet alone but in changing our response to our eating patterns as well as our attitude towards food. In this program we use all the keys in which to accomplish a weight loss program that works.

I have personally worked with helping many people lose pounds and inches following this program. The response and application has been very positive. Many clients were surprised at how well they were able to adhere to the program. They stated how they had tried many programs before but none of them decreased the cravings or gave them energy like The Slim Factor program does.

There will be some degree of adaptation that you must do. It takes dedication and strict adherence to all protocols. It is a strict 23 day program (followed by a 21 day consolidation process) which does make it attainable, allowing for transgressions afterwards, albeit in small doses, for this diet to be a success for you in the years following. You will lose weight and will maintain that weight loss afterwards.

The Slim Factor program has been adapted from Dr. A. T. W. Simeons', *Pounds and Inches* Program with some modern day adjustments. Simeons was a British doctor who had a clinic in Rome. He started his diet program in 1955 with people staying for 3-6 weeks in his infirmary. I am going to share his secret with you so you do not have to venture to an expensive retreat for six weeks. This program can be done in the comfort of your own home if you follow the program as given in the book.

Not only will the weight literally drop off from the hips, shoulders, thighs, and stomach, but you will have more energy and be more relaxed. You will look radiant. People will stop and take a double look at you. You will exude radiance. So many people told me it was not just the weight I had lost, but I looked 10 years younger, I looked alive, my eyes sparkled. The compliments astounded me. Everywhere I went people wanted to know my secret, well here it is, all in this book.

J.Dargan

WHY SOME PEOPLE ARE OVERWEIGHT, YET EAT VERY LITTLE, WHILE OTHERS CAN EAT ANYTHING THEY LIKE AND STILL NOT PUT ON WEIGHT?

This dilemma is one that I have had to address ever since I married my husband. It is not me that the biscuits and the chocolates have to be hidden from, it is him. He is able to eat whatever he likes without any consequences. We are both healthy eaters but the two of us had completely different metabolisms. I used to say that he would digest the food, and then once we were in bed, the calories would jump onto me by simply being beside him in the bed. It was so infuriating. I was denying myself biscuits and chocolates and not losing any weight and have him eating what he liked with nothing to show for it.

Even though I had a marginally better diet than my husband, he had more energy than me, blood pressure was within normal limits and cholesterol levels always came back fine. What was it that he had that I clearly did not? It is obvious that his body is in a constant fat burning mode, while mine was in a constant fat storage mode. His body knows when to stop storing fat, registering when it has enough fat stores. Thus his body rarely goes into fat storage mode. In order to fully understand this new phenomenon I am going to have to start with some technical talk which will open your mind up to a new possibility as to why you are having trouble losing weight. You will realise that there are other powers at play here and how you can overcome them and be the New, Slim You.

TESTIMONIES FROM CLIENTS DURING THE SLIM FACTOR PROGRAM:

It was a great feeling when I did not have to open my trouser button in order to get my trousers off. That had never happened before in my life. CM

Fat "blobs" on my legs that I had for years have now disappeared after the 21 day VLCD program. AN.

Everywhere I go people are asking me what I have done to myself, I look so fantastic. RL

I now jump out of bed in the morning full of energy. That has not happened in a long time. TT

Picking up the children from school is a new experience for me. The mothers stop talking and cannot stop looking at me. Of course they do not ask if I have lost weight but I do notice the look of envy in their eyes. JL

PART ONE

CHAPTER 1

INTRODUCING LEPTIN:
THE MESSENGER BETWEEN THE HYPOTHALAMUS AND THE FAT STORES.

Up until a few years ago, scientists believed that the fat tissue in our bodies was simply a metabolically inactive organ that served no purpose. When accumulated in excess it simply expanded your waist-line and other areas in the body with no other repercussions. In 1994, researchers at Rockefeller University made a discovery that disputed this belief and discovered that fat cells play a major role in our body's processes. They identified leptin as the hormone actually produced by fat tissue that signified satiety, the feeling of fullness, with the realization that fat cells played a major role in hormonal regulation.

We know now that leptin, a hormone, was only discovered recently in 1994. Leptin's role is to act as messenger between the hypothalamus and the fat stores. Leptin tells the hypothalamus in the brain that the body fat cells are full, or close to being filled, with fat (specifically triglycerides). This will then allow the body to stop absorbing fat from the food being eaten, but rather will start utilizing it, as well as burning any stored fat. In normal circumstances, when the body has stored enough fat, leptin sends messages to the hypothalamus saying enough fat has been stored and therefore, please, do not store any more. If our hypothalamus was working properly it would understand this message and stop storing any extra fat. Signals would be sent telling us to **stop eating**, that we are full, that we have had enough. But something seriously wrong is happening and the signals that we should be registering (telling us that we are full and to stop eating) are just not getting through to some people's brains.

LEPTIN SOME SIMPLE FACTS

Leptin is secreted predominantly by fat cells that influence energy expenditure and food intake in mammals. Leptin is released by fat cells and then enters the blood stream where it is delivered to the brain. After crossing the blood brain barrier, it travels to the hypothalamus where the hypothalamus registers how much fat is being stored in the body according to the amount of leptin that crossed the blood brain barrier. Leptin is highly regarded as being the principle modulator (that is, reduce body fat while enhancing lean body mass) of body weight and metabolism. It signals the hypothalamus on how much fat is being stored and assists in regulating food intake. Leptin plays a role in the body in how fat is metabolized once it is in the body from the intake of food as well as regulating hunger. Leptin actually facilitates the process of breaking down stored triglycerides in your fat cells into free fatty acids allowing them to be used for energy. If leptin was working correctly in your body you would be breaking down fat and not storing fat. It has often been referred to as the obese gene because as fat cells increase in the body there is a parallel increase in leptin levels.

Leptin regulates virtually all the hormones in the body. It contributes to the functioning, or if the case may be, malfunctioning, of the hypothalamus. Leptin's main job is to report back to the hypothalamus gland in the brain on the situation of fat content in the body. It acts centrally in the brain's hypothalamus to inhibit food intake and increase energy expenditure which results in loss of fat tissue mass and increase in lean muscle mass. Once the hypothalamus receives the signal from leptin that there is sufficient fat being stored in the body, metabolic rate increases and the brain now knows that it is safe for it to burn excess fat.

Leptin disposes of fat by up-regulating thermogenesis (generation of heat) and metabolic rate. In other words, leptin is communicating with your brain telling you when you should be hungry, when to eat and when to begin fat creation or combustion.

Low levels of leptin in the hypothalamus signals the body to eat more while high leptin levels tell the body to stop eating because you are full thus shutting down your appetite.

Leptin coordinates the metabolic, endocrine and behavioural responses to hunger. Its behaviour affects our emotions and our food cravings as well as weight loss and weight gain. It also plays a major role in the body's inflammatory processes.

Leptin acts on the brain stem which in turn acts on serotonin, a hormone that controls appetite and mood. It is the body's master hormone for weight regulation and basic survival. It also regulates other hormones including thyroid, sex, adrenal and pancreatic hormones. Without leptin, these hormones cannot function properly.

Leptin is important in the management of the entire endocrine system and its complex relationship between one hormone and another. When you get your leptin functioning properly it tends to rebalance everything such as the thyroid and the adrenal organs. Leptin's important functions are in, not only regulating body weight and metabolism, but also in reproductive function. It plays a vital role in controlling hypothalamic activity, which in turn regulates much of our body's autonomic functions.

Table 2: Leptin's major regulatory role

MAJOR REGULATORY ROLES OF LEPTIN

- Stimulates hunger when levels are deficient (low) in the brain.
- Suppresses appetite when levels are high in brain.
- Stress response.
- Fat burning and storage.
- Body temperature.
- Heart rate.
- Blood pressure.
- Reproductive behaviour.
- Bone growth.
- Regulate immunity.
- Blood sugar levels.
- Supports cognitive function.

WHAT HAPPENS WHEN LEPTIN LEVELS FALL?

When there are decreased levels of leptin in circulation this is giving a signal to the body that there is a deficiency in calorie intake and that it is not safe to break down fat stores but a need to store more fat in the body. This informs the body that it has to slow down metabolism, over-stimulate appetite (causing you to eat more) and increase fat deposits in the body. Instead of focusing on leptin's role as a satiety signal and thus causing the person to regulate their food intake, leptin's main role comes into play as a starvation hormone that signals calorie deficits. When food intake is low, metabolism slows down in an effort to reduce energy demands. Less intake of food only causes the body to stores its fat reserves.

With the discovery of decreased leptin levels (which occurs only in a very small percentage of obese people) being the blame on decreased metabolism and increased storage of fat stores, scientists and pharmaceutical companies presumed the answer here would be to administer leptin to overweight people and their weight loss would miraculously occur. Now, before you race out to buy leptin, do read on. Leptin is enormously complex in the way it interacts with the body's systems and glands. Put more leptin into the system and instead of fostering weight loss, it only causes "leptin resistance" making the body less able to shed excess fat and keep it off. Results were not as expected. People did not lose weight when given leptin, rather they gained weight. The next chapter explains what is happening to leptin in our bodies and how it affects our fat storage and metabolism. It is not a deficiency in leptin that obese or overweight people have, but rather, an overabundance in leptin that is not able to do its job properly.

SUMMARY OF CHAPTER ONE

Leptin:
- is a hormone responsible for telling the body when it should be storing fat and when it should be releasing fat stores, keeping your body trim with good muscle tone.
- facilitates the breakdown of stored triglycerides in your fat cells.
- is responsible for maintaining proper function of the hypothalamus.
- affects our emotions and emotional attachment to food.
- regulates the thyroid gland, adrenal gland and pancreatic hormones.
- plays a major role in inflammatory processes in the body.

If you are having trouble losing weight and maintaining weight loss, leptin is most probably not working correctly in your body. One aim of The Slim Factor Program is to get your hormone leptin working correctly in the body in order to perform the above functions correctly.

CHAPTER TWO

LEPTIN RESISTANCE: A WEIGHT LOSS NIGHTMARE

Fat cells make leptin. Leptin is secreted from white adipocytes (white fat cells) and levels correlate with adipose tissue mass. Leptin is released by fat cells and then enters the blood stream where it is delivered to the brain. After crossing the blood brain barrier, it travels to the hypothalamus where the hypothalamus registers how much fat is being stored in the body according to the amount of leptin that crossed the blood brain barrier.

Leptin is made by the body fat cells and when the body has more fat cells, this creates more leptin. The increased levels of leptin circulating can overwhelm the hypothalamus causing it to no longer respond to leptin in the proper way, instead it is telling the body to store fat. When there is higher than normal leptin levels in circulation your body tries to adjust its basal leptin levels. The set point for leptin is raised thus allowing for increased levels of leptin to be in circulation. With the increased levels of leptin in circulation the hypothalamus loses its sensitivity to leptin and does not respond to high leptin levels correctly. When the body has too much leptin circulating in the body, the leptin receptors in the hypothalamus become desensitized. It appears that the hypothalamus is oblivious to the amount of leptin in circulation.

Another mechanism that could be in play when you are leptin resistant, is that some leptin is not able to cross the blood brain barrier successfully, thus the hypothalamus registers low levels of leptin. The blood is saturated with leptin but very little is crossing the blood brain barrier. When the brain receives small amounts of leptin, it assumes that the body has correlating small amounts of fat cells. The brain does not properly register how much fat stores there are in the body with more fat cells being perceived as being needed in order to produce more leptin. Thus a vicious cycle further perpetuates. You sense hunger due to the fact that your hypothalamus is sending signals that you are not storing enough fat. This is due to the fact that it is registering low levels of leptin, despite the fact that there is actually an overabundance of leptin in circulation.

Overweight and obese people almost invariable have developed a resistance to leptin. What needs to happen is that the body needs to overcome this resistance in order to get the body back in shape. If you are leptin resistant, an increased amount of leptin will be needed in order to feel satisfied after a meal, resulting in more food being eaten, while at the same time, the body is burning LESS fat for fuel. What is happening here is the hypothalamus mis-believes that the body is starving, which causes the body to go into emergency mode creating a vicious cycle of telling the body it needs to store fat, storing fat in a body that has more than enough fat stores. DO I HAVE YOUR ATTENTION?

Table 3: Symptoms of leptin resistance

SYMPTOMS COMMONLY ASSOCIATED WITH LEPTIN RESISTANCE.
• Stress eating.
• Hypothyroid symptoms.
• Low energy.
• Excess abdominal fat.
• Insomnia or other sleep disorders.
• Late night eating.
• Feeling tired during the day.
• Cravings for sweet foods, breads, cereals, pasta, crackers, chips, potatoes, soda drinks, beer and wine.

When you are leptin resistant, your brain is unable to detect proper leptin levels circulating in the body, with a result of not knowing exactly how much fat is actually in storage. Your brain deludes itself into thinking that you are the perfect weight resulting in NOT telling your body to burn fat. What is even worse is that it could send incorrect signals that you are SHORT on calories causing you to eat more food.

Leptin resistance, in conjunction with insulin resistance, are often at the root of blood sugar imbalances with an overwhelming urge to eat more food. It desensitizes your taste buds to sugar and makes you crave more sweet food including carbohydrate foods. Leptin is the hormone that controls ghrelin. Ghrelin is the hormone that causes us to want to eat more. When leptin resistance occurs, ghrelin also becomes less responsive to food intake. Elevated ghrelin triggers strong feelings of hunger, slows your metabolism and reduces your ability to burn fat.

People, who are overweight, have trouble shedding fat and keeping it off, are most likely leptin resistant. Restoring healthy leptin function is the most important step towards establishing healthy endocrine balance no matter what your age. It can also help eliminate forever the kind of food cravings and constant hunger that prevent permanent weight loss. In the same manner of leptin resistant fat cells, insulin resistant muscle cells lose their responsiveness to insulin, glucose molecules are then blocked from entering muscle tissue, causing increased blood sugar levels. The liver senses this hyperglycaemia with the liver cells responding by breaking down the excess sugar molecules and transforming them into free fatty acids. The free fatty acids are then put into the bloodstream, and deposited throughout your body and stored wherever you tend to store adipose fat cells such as the stomach, hips, butt, and breasts. With the increased fat stores, leptin production is increased, and the cycle is never ending.

Stress, most people should be aware of, is one of the leading causes of insomnia and sleep deprivation. Did you also know that, the less sleep you get, the more leptin resistant you become? Sleep deprivation also increases the release of the hormone ghrelin which increases hunger and appetite. Thus, not getting enough sleep also is a major trigger for weight gain. With high levels of cortisol associated with stress, especially at night triggering insomnia, your body is not relaxing and repairing itself as it should be doing while you sleep. People with high cortisol levels circulating at night typically will wake around 2.00-3.00 in the morning and find it very difficult to get back to sleep. High cortisol levels also are responsible for triggering food cravings, especially for sweets as well as for salty foods causing you to eat uncontrollably leading to further weight gain.

The more sleep deprived you become due to stress, the more intolerant you become to stress. Adding to the fray at this point is that the increasing stress elevates the hormone ghrelin, causing you to eat more food.

When leptin resistance is controlled, allowing leptin to return to normal levels and function properly in our body, it tends to rebalance adrenals, thyroid and sex hormones. Restoring healthy leptin function is the most important step in establishing a healthy endocrine balance, **eliminating food cravings** and **eliminating constant hunger** that controls so many people preventing any successful weight loss. Your food cravings and increased eating are due to incorrect leptin functioning and **not** due to any incompetency on your part. At last the secret is out as to why you may crave for food or why you find it difficult to adhere to dietary programs.

For many people, the best diet and exercise program in the world will not work, nor will the best stress-reduction protocol, unless leptin resistance is addressed along with other important hormones that regulate appetite. Some people are more susceptible to problems with leptin levels than others. Many people who are trying to lose weight can find it a difficult process, even if they are eating smaller portions and exercising regularly. This is where overcoming leptin resistance comes into play and why The Slim Factor program works.

In people who are overweight, the problem is not low leptin levels, but rather, high leptin levels causing leptin resistance. Leptin levels in the blood are not properly being registered by the hypothalamus, causing the body to store more fat. The irony here is that with more fat stores being created, more leptin is being secreted with a vicious cycle that needs to be broken.

The most important issue that needs to be addressed is to get leptin levels to within normal range allowing the hypothalamus to work in its normal capacity.

SUMMARY OF CHAPTER TWO

- Leptin resistance is one of the main causes of obesity.
- Leptin is released from the fat cells into the blood stream where it crosses the blood brain barrier before it is registered by the hypothalamus.
- Leptin resistance needs to be addressed before any successful weight loss will be achieved.
- Stress and lack of sleep can both interfere with proper leptin function.

CHAPTER 3

WHY ARE PEOPLE LEPTIN RESISTANT?

Food without nutritional value (such as refined carbohydrates), foods containing high-fructose corn syrup and trans-fats, and other fake foods, send erroneous (incorrect) signals to the brain. The body interprets those signals as starvation, which makes the body burn fewer calories and store fat even in the presence of high leptin levels. When leptin is high, your satiety switch is broken. As a result, you gain weight, because you will be forever hungry and won't have control over your appetite.

Chronic overeating and frequent snacking may be one of the reasons, but not everyone who is leptin resistant should be labelled as chronic overeaters. Being leptin resistant can cause people to overeat as they are never truly satisfied after a meal.

1. High Fructose Corn Syrup (HFCS).

You may have easily been misled in believing that the fructose in high fructose corn syrup is a healthier alternative to sugar. I could write a whole book on the avoidance of high fructose corn syrup, also known as HFCS or simply corn syrup, as well as a whole list of alternative sugars, but will control myself at this point.

HFCS is made from corn syrup using enzymes to increase the fructose content. The fructose in HFCS is free, unbound fructose whereas fructose in fruit (more correctly to be referred to as levulose) is bound to other sugars. Fructose in fruit is surrounded by fibre, phytochemicals, vitamins, minerals and fatty acids. When fructose is extracted from its natural source and concentrated as a sweetener, it creates havoc on the body's metabolism. The fructose in HFCS is not able to be accessed for energy utilisation, but is converted into triglycerides and body fat. By not being used for energy utilisation this means that HFCS does not get used by the body at all for immediate energy, as opposed to sugar which is readily used by the body for its energy needs (whatever sugar is not used will be converted to fat).

All HFCS is immediately converted to triglycerides and body fat.

Fructose can raise triglyceride levels, increase the risk of heart disease as well as contributing to leptin resistance in the body. A study published in the Science Daily (2009), found that obese people who drank a fructose-sweetened drink with a meal had nearly 200% higher triglyceride levels than those who drank a glucose-sweetened drink with their meals. While I am not advocating glucose sweetened drinks at all, replacing a glucose drink with a fructose-sweetened drink is definitely not a better alternative.

Sugar, being a disaccharide, breaks down into two monosacchrides namely glucose and fructose. Small amounts of fructose in the diet increase production of glycogen (how sugar is stored in the body) as well as decrease the release of glucose into the bloodstream. Such a mechanism was once believed to be helpful for those suffering Type II diabetes. For diabetics it is important to control blood glucose and insulin levels to avoid complications. So, it would seem that a lack of glucose and insulin secretion from fructose consumption would be a good thing. However, insulin also controls leptin, so its release is necessary. Leptin tells your body to stop eating when it's full by signaling the brain to stop sending hunger signals. Since fructose doesn't stimulate glucose levels and insulin release, there's no increase in leptin levels or feeling of satiety. Fructose requires a different metabolic pathway than other carbohydrates because it basically skips glycolysis (normal carbohydrate metabolism). It then becomes material for fatty acid synthesis. This, combined with unstimulated leptin levels, is like opening the flood gates of fat deposition.

What happens then is that fructose is metabolized by the liver to free fatty acids and triglycerides. When large amounts of fructose are added to the diet it is rapidly converted into fatty acids which are then added to your fat stores or released into the bloodstream as triglycerides. The triglycerides bind with leptin thus interfering with leptin's ability to cross the blood brain barrier. You have to remember here that leptin has to first cross the blood brain barrier before it is able to reach the hypothalamus. If it is unable to reach the hypothalamus then the hypothalamus does not properly register the amount of leptin in circulation.

HFCS is rapidly converted to fatty acids and ultimately triglycerides (adding to fat stores in the body resulting in your getting fatter). The increased amount of triglycerides in the blood, bind with leptin and create large molecules that are unable to cross the blood brain barrier thus blocking leptin from getting into the hypothalamus.

Glucose provides "satiety" (feeling of being satisfied after a meal) signals whereas fructose does not due to the fact that it is unable to cross the blood-brain barrier. Also, fructose does not suppress ghrelin (the hunger hormone). So, when foods are sweetened with HFCS you will not feel satisfied due to signals not reaching the brain telling us that we have eaten enough, especially enough sugars.

You should always try to avoid high fructose corn syrup (HFCS) which can also be written as corn syrup, sucrose, dextrose, malto dextrose. Studies have shown that giving people yogurt sweetened with sugar did not eat as much as those who were fed artificially sweetened yogurt. The premise is that eating real sugar sets off a response that lets the body know that real calories are being consumed. In turn, the person feels satisfied after eating. Those that ate the artificially sweetened yogurt did not have that response of being satisfied with the amount of food being consumed. They ate more, which caused them to gain weight and body fat.

For more information on HFCS see Appendix #9 at the back of this book.

2. C-reactive Protein (CRP).

C-reactive protein is not normally found in the blood of healthy people. It appears after an injury, infection, or inflammation. The amount of CRP produced by the body varies from person to person, with individual's genetic makeup and lifestyle being the main contributors. Higher CRP levels tend to be found in individuals who are overweight and do not exercise, as well as in those who smoke, and have high blood pressure. Inflammation in fat tissue and blood vessels stimulates the production of CRP that disable leptin's ability to suppress appetite and speed metabolism. Individuals who are lean and athletic tend to have lower CRP levels.

A 2006 study conducted by researchers at the University of Pittsburgh showed that elevated levels of CRP inhibit leptin's role in controlling appetite.(K. Chen. 2006) The study showed CRP, in human blood interacts directly with serum leptin. CRP is a marker of systemic inflammation and predictor of cardiac risk. CRP is produced by the liver in response to factors released by fat cells. The study's major breakthrough was when it was discovered that human CRP binds with leptin and, in doing so, may prevent leptin from signalling satiety. CRP aggressively binds to leptin, creating a large molecule that cannot cross the blood-brain barrier. Therefore the leptin never gets to the hypothalamus, and the hypothalamus incorrectly assumes the body has low levels of leptin in circulation (and therefore low in fat cells), thus the body never gets the message to stop eating.

One theory here is that weight gain leads to increased leptin with the body initiating an inflammatory response by releasing CRP which then binds with leptin in order to limit damage from high leptin levels, that the body does this as a defence mechanism!

As inflammation levels increase, CRP increases also. You should also be aware that inflammation is actually generated by excess fat! This in turn leads to more weight gain which causes more leptin. This cycle needs to be stopped and fast!

3. Hydrogenated (transfats) foods.

Hydrogenated fats are man-made processed fats, which are made from liquid oil. When you add hydrogen to liquid vegetable oil and then add pressure, a hydrogenated fat is the result. Hydrogenated fats are also called transfats. Hydrogenated fats pose a high risk of heart disease. Not only do they raise total cholesterol levels, but they also deplete good cholesterol (HDL), which helps protect against heart disease. Hydrogenated fats do the same thing in our bodies that bacon grease does to kitchen sinks. Over time, they can clog the blood vessels that feed the heart and brain, which can lead to heart attack or stroke. High amounts of triglycerides in the body bind with leptin making it harder for leptin to cross the blood brain barrier causing a decreased transport of leptin across the blood brain barrier.

Hydrogenated fats compete with good fats, so it's important to minimize the intake of hydrogenated fats as well as consuming enough good fats (see Appendix # 3: Supplements). Good fats raise your HDL or "good cholesterol" which is responsible for delivering your bad cholesterol (LDL), to the liver where it is broken down and excreted from the body. Good fats also help the body to respond better to leptin and thus increase your fat burning metabolism.

Leptin's ability to work in its correct mode is hindered when it is bound. Both triglycerides and C-reactive protein bind to leptin thus creating a molecule that is too large to cross the blood brain barrier. Leptin is therefore unable to make its way to the hypothalamus. The hypothalamus then incorrectly registers that the body has no fat stores due to low leptin levels reaching the hypothalamus. Thus it sends signals to the body to store more fat.

4. Monosodium glutamate (MSG)

Monosodium glutamate (MSG), in its many forms, along with aspartic acid, has been shown to cause hypothalamic lesions, which in turn leads to obesity. Animal studies indicate that MSG can induce hypothalamic lesions and leptin resistance, possibly influencing energy balance, leading to increased fat stores. The study found that by eating MSG, it is very likely to damage the hypothalamic regulation of your appetite. (Ka He, Liancheng Zhao et al, 2008) The damage to the hypothalamus caused by MSG is a major reason why some people are leptin resistant.

MSG can be a nightmare for those trying to lose weight. It is found in so many foods, under many different names in order to disguise its presence in foods, that the only fool proof way to avoid MSG is to avoid processed foods as much as possible. Although Chinese restaurants get most of the bad press of food containing MSG, you would be surprised just how MSG is getting into your diet without you realising it. Manufacturers can correctly claim that there is no MSG in their products as long as the MSG is a constituent of an ingredient in the product. Some fancy names for MSG include calcium caseinate, glutamic acid, textured protein, autolysed yeast extract or simply E621.

Foods with MSG can make us addicted to such foods in much the same way nicotine makes cigarette smokers hooked. When was the last time you stopped with one potato chip?

5. Aspartamine

Aspartame, the artificial sweetener found in most diet drinks, has also been found to cause lesions on the hypothalamus. Aspartamine is an excitotoxin that energises the nerves in the brain. Nerves do need to be stimulated for normal functioning of the brain, but the presence of excitotoxins will not allow the nerves to shut down. If nerve cells remain excited they eventually die causing hypothalamic lesions. This is another reason for a low functioning hypothalamus with impaired responses to leptin levels in the body.

Lesions on the hypothalamus cause the hypothalamus to not function properly. Hence, leptin levels are not being properly registered by the hypothalamus and signals from the hypothalamus are not accurate.

6. Carbohydrate foods.

The major source of food offenders triggering leptin resistance are carbohydrate foods and their subsequent blood sugar surges. They trigger leptin dysregulation and hormone imbalance, create blood sugar disorders, produce cravings and interfere with normal insulin behaviour. Examples of such foods are bread, potatoes, pasta, cereal, rice, and other starchy vegetables, as well as wine and beer.

Carbohydrate foods, no matter if they are simple or complex, once digested, are broken down to glucose. Insulin is released in response to the increase of glucose in the blood. The more the blood is flooded with glucose, the more insulin will be produced. Excess insulin causes the body to store the excess sugars as fat. With a high carbohydrate diet (and subsequent high insulin being released), the body is in a fat storage mode. Unless you are an athlete training 4-7 days a week and rapidly breaking down carbohydrates for instant energy and glycogen replacement, most of the carbohydrate foods eaten will ultimately be converted to fat for storage by the body.

Something for you to think about: When a steam train is in full throttle it rapidly uses up the wood and coal put into the furnace. If the train is ambling along the track, the valve is closed somewhat and very little wood and coal is used. If you keep filling up the furnace with more wood and coal while the train is moving slowly, then the furnace will overflow. A train's furnace is solid and cannot expand, but keep filling your body with carbohydrates, with little or no exercise, and you will expand!

Everybody needs a certain level of carbohydrates for energy, but whatever is not utilised by the body for energy will be stored as fat in the body. With the increase in fat cells, more leptin is produced.

7. Other sugar substitutes.

Alternative sugars, include sucralose, Splenda, aspartamine, maltose, basically the list is endless. No matter how they are disguised, they are a poison to the body and need to be addressed. These are all man made under ultra high processing that over taxes the hypothalamus and makes people fat. More fat cells lead to more leptin being released.

We are eating far too many sugars in our society, allowing ourselves to be deluded that we are not, simply due to the way manufacturers find ingenious ways to disguise the names for sugars. Basically, you should be getting your sugar kicks in the natural form, and that is from fruits and honey. By all means, we all need sweetness in life, but keep treats to a minimum and you will enjoy them more and your body will certainly thank you for it.

8. Other reasons.

Exposure to toxins, candida overgrowth, prescription drugs such as steroids and antibiotics, all contribute to liver dysfunction and weight gain, creating larger fat cells filled with even more leptin. This increase in leptin reports to the hypothalamus thus overloading the gland's leptin receptors to a point of desensitization in the process.

More fat cells create more leptin.

WHY DOES THE BODY ALLOW LEPTIN RESISTANCE TO OCCUR?

Believe it or not, but our bodies were actually designed for leptin, as well as, insulin resistance. In times past, people feasted in the summer and early autumn when food was plentiful, to store fat for winter when food was scarce. Summer was the time to eat as much as possible, especially carbohydrates (albeit mostly in the form of fruit and honey) so that enough weight would be gained to make it through the lean winter months. In fact, our survival as a civilization depended on this biochemistry which does make sense.

In modern day society, winter no longer means hibernating away. There is a constant supply of food with no shortages during the winter months thanks to air travel. Artificial lights have us awake till late, in both summer and winter. In winter houses are heated and we are eating the same amount of endless carbohydrates in both winter and summer.

We are in a constant "store fat for winter" scenario which seriously needs to be addressed. We also need to learn how to cook from basics and rely less on processed foods.

We are also eating too many calories for the level of activity we are achieving each day. Daily caloric counts should, as a rough guide, be as follows: (based on female 145lb, 5"5')

1. Work in an office with very little exercise: 1600 calories/day
2. Active at work and do some light exercise or long walks: 1900 calories/day
3. Very active at work and home, exercising several times a week: 2140 calories/day
4. Very intense work and home activity, participating in physical sports every day: 2380 calories/day.

Table 4: Complications due to increased leptin levels.

COMPLICATIONS ASSOCIATED WITH INCREASED LEPTIN LEVELS
• Obesity. • Hypertension. • Hyper-lipidaemia. • Metabolic syndrome. • Psoriasis. • Arthritis. • Inflammatory conditions. • Increased risk of chronic heart disease and cancer.

FLOW SHEET OF LEPTIN RESISTANCE

Summary of Chapter Three.

Diagram of how messages are not correctly getting through to the hypothalamus. Broken line denotes messages not being able to penetrate the blood brain barrier. What then happens is that the brain is sending out incorrect messages, telling the body that it needs to be storing more fat due to the fact that it misbelieves that the body does not have enough fat stores.

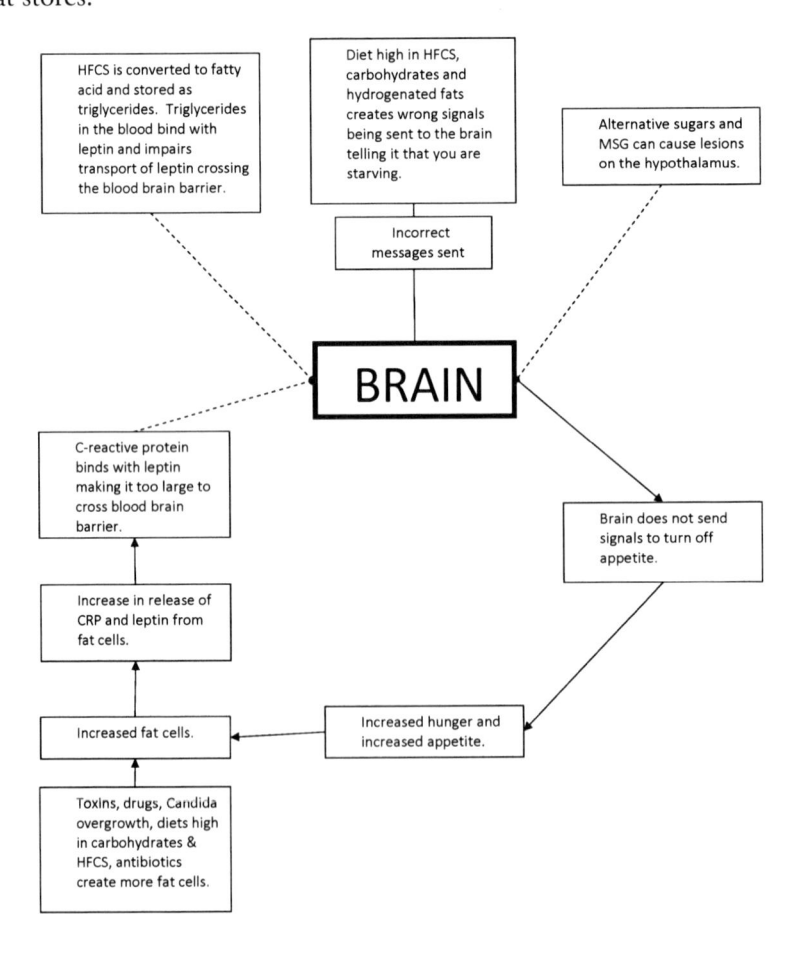

- HFCS is converted to fatty acid and stored as triglycerides. Triglycerides in the blood bind with leptin and impairs transport of leptin crossing the blood brain barrier.
- Diet high in HFCS, carbohydrates and hydrogenated fats creates wrong signals being sent to the brain telling it that you are starving.
- Alternative sugars and MSG can cause lesions on the hypothalamus.
- Incorrect messages sent

BRAIN

- C-reactive protein binds with leptin making it too large to cross blood brain barrier.
- Increase in release of CRP and leptin from fat cells.
- Increased fat cells.
- Toxins, drugs, Candida overgrowth, diets high in carbohydrates & HFCS, antibiotics create more fat cells.
- Increased hunger and increased appetite.
- Brain does not send signals to turn off appetite.

CHAPTER FOUR

THE DIENCEPHALON
INTRODUCING DR. A.T.W. SIMEONS

Dr. Simeons committed 40 years of his life seeking to unlock the mystery to obesity in people. His research included thyroid, pituitary and adrenal glands, as well as the pancreas and the gallbladder. Dr. Simeons, author of Pounds and Inches: A new approach to Obesity, (1971) through years of research, was able to pinpoint the key to obesity problem lies within the part of the brain referred to as the diencephalon. The diencephalon is a complex of structures that includes the thalamus as well as the hypothalamus. He concluded that the hypothalamus in particular was compromised and was at the root of the problem in relation to obesity.

Dr. Simeons was able to deduce that if obesity is always due to one specific diencephalon deficiency, then, in order to overcome obesity, there is the need to correct this deficiency. After much research, he found that by administering hCG in overweight people they lost their increased appetites and bodies were reshaped due to the loss of body fat. hCG was assisting in **opening the abnormal, secure reserves of fat** and actually getting them **mobilised** and e**liminated** from the body. When hCG is taken, in combination with a low calorie diet, it recalibrates the hypothalamus and helps unlock fat deposits which are then used as fuel in the body.

THE HYPOTHALAMUS

The hypothalamus, often referred to as the master gland, is responsible for fat storage in the body. Dr. Simeons believed that over-eating is the **results of a metabolic disorder**, and not its cause, disputing the commonly believed theory that over eating causes obesity.

Within the hypothalamus is the satiety centre that regulates appetite. It is controlled by two chemicals that stimulate the hypothalamus to increase metabolism, decrease appetite and increase insulin to deliver energy to cells rather than it being stored as fat. The hypothalamus gland modulates the thyroid, adrenals, fat storage, and more importantly, your metabolic rate. It also controls hunger, temperature, emotions, thirst, and fatigue as well as develop the reproductive organs during puberty.

When the hypothalamus is not functioning properly (as discussed in Chapter Three), the body will store abnormal fat instead of burning it. With a low functioning hypothalamus you can crave food which is not properly utilised by the body. Instead, it is stored in abnormal fat reserves that are very difficult to access and be removed. An imbalance of the hypothalamus can cause constant hunger, low metabolism, and accumulation of excessive and abnormal fat deposits on the body. In most over weight and obese people their hypothalamus is impaired.

When normal functioning of the hypothalamus is compromised, fat will increase whether you eat excessively, normally or minimally. No amount of dieting or exercise will allow the stored fat reserves to budge. In order for the stored fat reserves to be released, increase the body's metabolism and reduce hunger pangs, the hypothalamus must be reset. This is one of the aims of The Slim Factor program, the resetting of the hypothalamus.

Once the hypothalamus is repaired, then the body is able to nurture other glands such as the thyroid and the adrenals.

Table 5: Causes of Hypothalamic Impairment

WHAT CAUSES HYPOTHALAMUS FUNCTION TO BE IMPAIRED?
• Foods contaminated with man-made chemicals (found in most, if not all, processed foods) such as **MSG and aspartame** as discussed in Chapter three. • Increased levels of circulating **leptin** as discussed in Chapter three • Stress. • Trauma. • Cycles of fasting and bingeing. • Diet of highly refined, low-fibre food..

THE SLIM FACTOR IN ACTION

In order for your body to stop storing fat and start working in fat burning mode the following needs to be addressed.

1. First and foremost what needs to be done, to tackle any overweight problem, is to heal the hypothalamus. First step is to stop any intake of substances that may cause lesions to the hypothalamus (such as aspartamine).

Need to heal the hypothalamus of any lesions by stopping substances that interfere with proper hypothalamic functioning.

2. The next step is to unblock any bound leptin that is unable to cross the blood brain barrier. Need to decrease any bound leptin levels in circulation.

Need to unbind the leptin from C-reactive protein and triglycerides in order to allow leptin to cross the blood brain barrier and thus enter the hypothalamus.

3. It is crucial in any diet to rid the body of abnormal fat.

Need to decrease fat cells in the body.

Once the amount of fat cells is reduced and eliminated, then the amount of leptin, C-reactive protein and triglycerides begins to return to normal levels. Only then will the process of healing the disconnected communication between the fat stores and the hypothalamus can occur. When this communication is restored and working harmoniously in the body, the hypothalamus will once again reign in the role of prompting the body to decrease food intake through appetite and increase energy output thus burning any extra calories eaten.

This is where The Slim Factor program is so successful and where most other weight reduction programs fail. All three issues addressed as above are addressed on The Slim Factor Program. Once these are achieved then the hypothalamus is able to work in its correct capacity. If the body does not eliminate the abnormal fat stores, the high levels of leptin circulating in the body will keep the body forever locked in leptin resistance mode. The Slim Factor Program also addresses the issue of healing the hypothalamus. In other diet programs the hypothalamus will continue to allow the body to store fat and keep the appetite elevated once any program is finished. This does not happen on The Slim Factor Program once the hypothalamus has been reset. Once your hypothalamus is reset the body will know how much fat there is in the body and will not incorrectly store fat.

AIM OF SLIM FACTOR PROGRAM

- Decrease leptin levels to normal, healthy ranges.
- Decrease triglycerides and C-reactive protein levels thus allowing leptin to be unbound and able to cross the blood brain barrier.
- Heal the hypothalamus.
- Healthy, unbound leptin levels and a healed hypothalamus lead to long term weight control.

SUMMARY OF CHAPTER FOUR

- First step is to heal the hypothalamus: the master gland.
- Leptin levels need to return to normal range (as well as unbound) in order for the hypothalamus to perform efficiently and to maximum capacity.
- Need to move the body from a fat-storage mode into a fat burning mode.
- Need to overcome diencephalon deficiency in order to overcome obesity.
- Increased circulating leptin and a diet high in processed foods are two major reasons why hypothalamic function may be impaired.
- Leptin needs to be unbound from circulating C-reactive protein and triglycerides in order to be able to cross the blood brain barrier and be registered by the hypothalamus.

CHAPTER FIVE

ABNORMAL FATS VS NORMAL FATS

There are three types of fat in our body.

1. Structural
2. Essential
3. Non-essential

The first type of body fat is the **Structural fat** which fills the gaps between various organs. Structural fat also performs important functions such as bedding the kidneys in soft elastic tissue, protecting the coronary arteries and keeping the skin smooth and taut. It also provides the springy cushion of hard fat under the bones of the feet, without which we would be unable to walk.

The second type of fat is the **Essential** fat reserves. This is the normal reserve of fuel used when the body is faced with immediate dietary insufficiencies such as regular low calorie diets. Such normal reserves are localized all over the body. Fat is a substance which packs the highest caloric value into the smallest space so that normal reserves of fuel for muscular activity and the maintenance of body temperature can be most economically stored in this form.

Both types of fat, structural and essential, are normal, and even if the body stocks them to capacity this can never be called obesity.

The third type of fat is entirely abnormal and is **Non-essential.** It is the accumulation of this fat from which the overweight person suffers. This abnormal fat is also a potential reserve of fuel, but unlike the normal reserves it is **not available** to the body in a nutritional emergency or during most diet programs. This third type of fat causes the body to be misshapen and is the causative factor in health problems. It is the unused store house of energy. This type of fat is the chief cause of obesity due to its ability to slow down the metabolic rate as well as being very difficult to remove. It is also a **major** source of leptin.

It is the abnormal fat, secured away in the body, which this program targets. In order to lose weight, the non-essential fat stores need to be opened and removed from the body.

Under normal dieting programs, the fat which will be released will only be the first two fat reserves as explained above, namely the structural fat and essential fat reserves, as well as muscle and water. The abnormal fat reserves are rarely tapped into to be removed. <u>These are the fat reserves that need to be removed and will be removed on The Slim Factor program.</u>

Our weight loss protocol centres on healing and resetting the hypothalamus. This program will allow your hypothalamus to be healed of any lesions, as well as reset and function correctly. Leptin levels will also return to normal levels and thus function in their correct capacity.

What happens in most regular diets is that fat is taken from the much needed structural and essential fat stores leaving you looking haggard. Have you ever found yourself with very sore heels during or after dieting? That is because while you were limiting your calorie intake the body was breaking down structural fat in order to fuel the body. One example of this would be the breaking down of hard fat under the bones of the feet leaving you walking on very little cushioning in that area.

For any diet to work, it is crucial that it has to rid the body of abnormal fat. Only once the number of fat cells is reduced and eliminated, can the amount of leptin begin to return to normal levels. Only then will the process of healing the disconnected communication between the fat stores and the hypothalamus actually take place. When this communication is restored and working harmoniously in the body, the hypothalamus will once again reign in the role of prompting the body to decrease food intake through decreasing appetite and increasing energy output by increasing metabolism.

This is where The Slim Factor program is so successful and that most other weight reduction programs fail. If the body does not eliminate the abnormal fat stores, the high levels of leptin circulating in the body will keep the body forever locked in leptin resistance mode. The hypothalamus will continue to allow the body to store fat and keep the appetite elevated.

THYROID MYTHS

It is true that the thyroid gland controls the rate at which body-fuel is consumed. Many articles are written about the benefits of kelp, for example, to reduce weight by increasing the body's metabolism. Simeons argued that a misconception exists in that when administering thyroid gland medication, or kelp etc, to an overweight or obese person, their abnormal fat deposits could be burned up more rapidly. The result is a disappointing NO due to the fact that the abnormal fat deposits are tightly packed away and therefore take no part in the body's energy turnover. Any thyroid medication or herbal remedy aimed at the thyroid only forces the body to consume its structural and essential fat reserves, which may be already depleted in obese patients, without touching the packed away abnormal fat deposits. Any weight loss that occurs whilst on thyroid medication will be at the expense of essential fat, and not abnormal fat deposits.

With leptin resistance, the thyroid function is suppressed causing many people to suffer low metabolism. This can be attributed not to any intrinsic deficiency of the thyroid gland, but rather to a lack of diencephalon stimulation of the thyroid gland via the anterior pituitary lobe. What I am trying to relay here is that, low metabolism is not directly due to a low thyroid condition but to low stimulation of the thyroid. Many people mistakenly concentrate on their weight gain as being due to a thyroid condition. This may be true for some, but for most people once the diencephalon area is working in its proper capacity, so too does the thyroid gland. A good analogy of this would be as follows:

A water tower is responsible for transferring water to a storage container from which water is drawn from for everyday use. One day there is no water to be drawn from the storage container. If the water tower is somewhat blocked then no amount of work performed on the storage container will produce water. The water tower needs to be addressed first and then the storage container will work. At first it may have appeared that the problem was with the storage container, but it was actually from the water tower.

On The Slim Factor program, thyroid function will be augmented thus regaining its proper working capacity once the hypothalamus is up and running properly.

SUMMARY OF CHAPTER FIVE

- There are three types of body fat. The aim of The Slim Factor program is to remove the Non-Essential fat stores only.
- The Slim Factor program centres on healing and resetting the hypothalamus.
- Abnormal (non essential) fat stores are never accessed for energy by the body under the influence of thyroid medication.

CHAPTER SIX

WHAT IS hCG?

hCG, human chorionic gonadotropin, is a substance produced by the placenta during pregnancy. It is also found in low levels in healthy men as well as healthy, non-pregnant women. Low levels are secreted from the gonadotrophin cells of the pituitary. (R. Sood 2005)

Everyone has hCG circulating in their body from birth. Chemicals in our foods and Candida yeast overgrowth are two causes of creating very low levels of hCG in the body. Dr. Simeons found that hCG signals the body to mobilise the abnormal fat reserves when given in conjunction with a very low caloric diet (VLCD) and tricks the body as though it were dealing with a near emergency starvation situation. Decreased lipogenesis (a decrease in the creation of fat stores) and enhanced lipolysis (the breakdown of fat stores), stimulated by the VLCD and intake of hCG, leads to a decrease of fat deposits in the body. hCG also enhances normal leptin activity which is another factor attributing to decreasing leptin resistance.

Through its hypothalamic action, hCG decreases lipogenesis in body fat tissue. Once taken, hCG accumulates in the hypothalamic region. Endorphin content in hCG accounts for modulation of hypothalamic area thus the improvement in mood whilst on this program. Selective lipolysis of specific fat regions in the body modulates body contour.

In plain English, what this means is that hCG decreases the making of fat in the body at the same time increasing the breakdown of fat which is then removed by the body. It also improves leptin interaction within the hypothalamus thus decreasing leptin resistance. Once hCG levels increase in the hypothalamus it gives you a feeling of euphoria, which accounts for the feel good factor associated with this program. hCG also contributes to selective breakdown of body fats hence giving you the body shape you are striving for.

Current research is proving to link how hCG and leptin might be interacting to signal the same receptor sites in the hypothalamus. Research on this interaction is too new to explain exactly how it works, but it is clear that hCG and leptin influence one another. There is also the influence that leptin places on insulin leading to an indirect response between insulin and hCG. These protein hormones (insulin and leptin) both share the same properties in that over exposure of one leads to resistance. Leptin resistance leads to storage of too much fat while insulin resistance leads to abnormal blood sugar metabolism and subsequent storage of fat.

The Slim Factor program is unique in that it allows for the release of fat cells from abnormal fat stores into the bloodstream and therefore used as fuel for the body thus allowing you to subsist more on your stored fat than from what you are eating. The abnormal fat stores that are released are due to the administration of hCG. Without hCG these abnormal fat stores are not normally available for fuel. This is the downfall of most diets; the abnormal fat stores are not being properly unlocked and broken down. hCG encourages the hypothalamus to burn non-essential fat, even after the strict 21 day program is finished.

It is important to note that The Slim Factor program engages non-essential fat first, leaving structural and essential fat intact. Not only are they being broken down in this program, but they are actually reduced and eliminated from the body. That's right, fat cells gone forever. The weight loss comes from loss of abnormal fat and does not strip the body of much needed muscle, vitamins and minerals that are essential in maintaining good health while, at the same time, releasing excessive amounts of fat-stored nutrients into the blood stream to be absorbed by the body.

HOMEOPATHIC hCG.

Homeopathy is a healing modality based on the emerging science of energy medicine that imprints the energy of a substance without using the actual physical substance. The body is able to read the information and create the desired outcome. I have successfully used homeopathy in my practise as well as treating my family. It is a safe modality with none of the major side effects plaguing people every day when using pharmaceutical medicines.

Taken in very small doses, hCG aids the body in burning its non-essential (abnormal fat), which is usually found in excess in our stomach, back, butt, hips, thighs, and underside of arms. Under the influence of hCG, fat is excreted from your body cells, in which it is stored in fatty tissue. By using hCG homeopathic drops, the body begins to consume its own abnormal fat reserves. Taking the drops under the tongue allows for the hCG remedy to be rapidly absorbed by the body. It triggers the body to provide a constant flow of "food" received from the fat that your body is breaking down and using. When these cells are empty, the body breaks down the cellular structure and absorbs it. Yes, fat cells are broken down and removed, forever!

Homeopathic hCG encourages healthy leptin behaviour during The Slim Factor program. It also encourages long term good leptin behaviour which appears to protect from rebound weight gain long after the very low calorie diet is finished. hCG is what triggers the hypothalamus to mobilize stored fat into the bloodstream to be used as "food". It is believed to reset your metabolism and to protect your body's good fat and keep muscle tissue from breaking down (which occurs in other low calorie diets without the use of hCG).

Taking the hCG diet drops will cause your hypothalamus (which controls many of the bodies functions such as hunger, metabolism, etc.) to work at resetting your metabolism, so that when you complete the diet, the weight will stay off. The hypothalamus will then continually send signals to release stored fat reserves thus allowing you not to hold onto the stores.

SUMMARY OF CHAPTER SIX

- hCG is a hormone found naturally in the body.
- hCG is not attributed to decreasing any storage of fat in the body, rather it increases the release of fat stores from abnormal fat reserves.
- hCG helps give you a sense of euphoria from its endorphin (feel good factor) content.
- hCG enhances leptin activity allowing it to not be so resistant in the body.
- Homeopathic hCG is the safest way to take hCG.

Table 6: Lipogenesis vs lipolysis

Lipogensisis the process of making fat in the body.
Lipolysis is the breakdown of fats in the body for energy.

Table 7: Current diseases that improve while taking hCG:

CURRENT DISEASES THAT IMPROVE WHILE TAKING HCG:
Diabetes with decreased need for medication.*
Rheumatism with decreased need for medication.*
Cholesterol levels decrease.
Uric acid levels decrease with gout sufferers.
Blood pressure decreases.
Peptic ulcers heal.
Improvement in psoriasis, fingernails, hair and varicose ulcers.
Normalises thyroid function allowing for decrease or cessation of treatment.*
(* always under supervision)

CHAPTER SEVEN

OBJECTIVES OF THE SLIM FACTOR DIETARY PROGRAM

The objectives of The Slim Factor program is to restore leptin sensitivity (resistance) and heal hypothalamic lesions allowing for proper functioning of the hypothalamus allowing you to **burn fat for fuel**.

In order to achieve the weight loss you desire the following issues need to be, and will be, addressed.

- Fat cells need to be decreased in number in order to decrease leptin and C-reactive protein levels.
- Triglyceride levels need to be decreased in order to increase the transport of leptin across the blood brain barrier.
- Leptin needs to be unbound in order to cross the blood brain barrier.
- The hypothalamus needs to be restored to its optimum working capacity.
- Decrease on the reliance of foods that send erroneous messages to the hypothalamus.
- Signals from the brain need to be turned back on letting you get the correct signals that you are satisfied and not in a constant mode of hunger.

Once leptin sensitivity is restored, your cells will also become more sensitized to other hormones allowing them to work in their proper capacity. When leptin resistance is controlled and thus allowing leptin to function properly in our body, it tends to rebalance adrenals, thyroid and sex hormones. Restoring healthy leptin function is the most important step in establishing a healthy endocrine balance, eliminating food cravings and constant hunger that controls so many people thus preventing any successful weight loss.

You may be confused with some of the literature at this point. While it may not be important to fully understand the mechanics of The Slim Factor program, what you should be aware of is that this program works. You will lose the weight you want to lose, you will feel great, you will exude radiance, your clothes will fit you better than ever before and people will want to know your secret.

The 21 VLCD days in Phase One is teaching your body to burn fat instead of sugar, hence why no starch or carbohydrates are allowed. The 21 days in the Phase Two (Maintenance Phase) is a gradual introduction of starches and sugars. During this time the body's set point is set to a new lower level allowing you to maintain your weight loss once you have finished the program.

THE SLIM FACTOR PROGRAM.

<u>ONE CYCLE IS COMPRISED OF TWO PHASES</u>.

Phase One consists of two steps:
1. 2 Days: Loading Phase
2. 21 Very Low Calorie Diet (VLCD) days

Phase Two involves one step:
1. 21 Maintenance days

If you only need to lose 15 pounds (7 kg) or less, then only one application of Phase One of The Slim Factor program is required. This is then followed by Phase Two: 21 Maintenance Days.

The VLCD (Phase One: Step 2) never lasts less than 21 days, even if you only need to lose five pounds. In order for the program to be successful, the hypothalamic lesions will take three weeks to heal allowing the hypothalamus to return to its **normal working capacity** and **resetting your body's metabolism**. This is also the time needed for triglyceride and C-reactive levels to decrease and halt the attraction to leptin, thus allowing leptin to more easily pass the blood brain barrier.

If you require losing more pounds after completing Phase One, then you may continue with a second or even more applications of Phase One. You should always take a break for a couple of days, to a week, before instigating Phase One again. If you are going to take a break for longer than one week, then you must first complete Phase Two straight after Phase One to make sure your body's metabolism has reset properly.

You may return to Phase One whenever you wish. Some people like to do two cycles and then have a break for a month or two. Certainly no more than three cycles should be attempted in a row as this is too long to adhere to such a strict regime. Phase Two is very important and many people underestimate how hard it may be to adhere to.

hCG can be used safely, but as with most programs regarding your health or diet, you should always consult your doctor before starting any new diet or health program, including this program.

The diet, used in conjunction with hCG, must not exceed 500-550 calories per day, and the way these calories are made up is of utmost importance. For instance, if a banana is eaten instead of an apple, you may not be getting any extra calories, but you will also not lose weight. There are a number of foods, particularly fruits and vegetables, which have the same or even lower caloric values than those listed as permissible, and yet it has been found that they interfere with the regular loss of weight. It is also important to remember that you must receive at least 500 calories a day. There may be some days that you do not feel hungry (crazy as it may sound but true), but it is important to keep track of all calories in a day and make sure you are reaching 500 calories. If you do not then you may be putting your body into starvation mode and the body will no longer source your fat for fuel with the result of the body keeping its fat locked safely away in storage during such conditions.

Weight loss can be different for different people. Some have a steady two pounds per day while others may lose nothing for two days, then lose five pounds on the third day. Up to two pound per day can be lost, depending on the amount of fat in reserve to be lost. Every person loses the weight at different rates varying between half to three pounds per day. The most average weight loss is between one to two pounds per day. Most people seem to lose ten percent of their body weight during Phase One. Urinary output (passing of water) can be rather rapid in the first couple of days. I found myself going to the toilet three times a night but this will also relax a bit as the day's progress.

HOW DOES THE SLIM FACTOR PROGRAM WORK?

The Slim Factor program works by combining a VLCD (Very Low Calorie Diet) with hCG. Under the influence of hCG, the body begins to consume its own abnormal fat reserves, quickly but safely, because it is natural and does exactly what it is designed to do which is to convert fat to energy. The body will only release the abnormal fat reserves after it has burned up the consumed calories ingested. Although you may be concerned with your ability to survive on a VLCD (500 calories per day), what you may fail to remember is that for every pound of fat that will be released from your body, it is equal to 3500 calories being released from your fat cells. Therefore your body is NOT functioning on only the 500 calories per day that you eat, but ALSO on the 1,500-4,000 calories per day that you are converting from your fat reserves giving the body much needed energy and nutrition.

Weight loss on The Slim Factor program will only be as successful as you taking control of your life and making some serious changes once you have finished the program. You were over-weight in the first instance due to incorrect food choices, either intentionally or unintentionally. This program will see a life-long success rate if you adhere to the whole protocol and adjust your diet afterwards. It does not mean that you can eat all the biscuits, chocolates and ice-cream simply because you have re-programmed your body. Eating too much of the foods that made you leptin resistant in the first place will only make you leptin resistant again.

Remember, that you are losing inches and not just pounds. It is important to look at your weight loss success overall when you have completed the program.

VERY LOW CALORIE DIET VS VERY LOW CALORIE DIET WITH hCG.

Cutting back on your daily caloric intake and fat consumption will help you lose weight. However, just because you drop pounds, does not mean that you are losing the abnormal fat you are trying to lose and keep off. Typically when the body is placed on a very low calorie diet it will initially react to oppose the change. The effect is that the cellular metabolism will slow down and the body will actually store fat and first decrease its muscle mass. When a person goes on a low calorie diet **without** the hCG drops, the body goes into starvation mode, or as commonly known, a metabolic state. This causes the body to hold on to, and even build up, its abnormal fat reserves while seeking to sustain itself on lean muscle mass and essential fat reserves, which protect vital organs and bones. You will also be tired and look haggard. You will not have energy to do your usual daily activities.

By adding hCG to your diet program, excess unhealthy fat is targeted first and is mobilized for energy. What can't be used for energy is then simply eliminated. A low calorie diet in conjunction with hCG is essential because it prevents an instant restoration of the emptied fat cells. This is why hCG works. It maintains your muscle mass by getting rid of the fat deposits. Due to the fat stores being released you will have an abundance of energy as well as you will look and feel great throughout the program.

SUMMARY OF CHAPTER SEVEN

- One cycle consists of two phases.
- Phase One may be undertaken one to three times before Phase Two is implemented.
- Phase Two is to be done only once per cycle.
- Phase Two is just as important as Phase One. It is not to be ignored and must be implemented when you plan to no longer maintain the VLCD.
- Phase Two is to begin on Day 24 of your last Slim Factor cycle.
- Once you have completed Phase Two you may do more cycles if you need to lose more weight after taking a break for at least one month.

CHAPTER EIGHT

STARTING THE PROGRAM
SIMPLE TASKS BEFORE YOU START THE PROGRAM

- Write down on paper what are your goals in doing this program. You may be doing the program to simply lose weight or you may be doing it to relieve your body of the aches and pains you are now suffering from. By writing down your goals you will be able to use this vision in order to maintain the strict adherence to the VLCD.
- Clear out your cupboards if you feel biscuits and chocolates may be too tempting to have in easy reach.
- Make out menu plans for the week.
- Freeze meals.
- Have snacks handy both home and work such as your fruit.
- Seek out positive people.
- Reward yourself periodically: soak in a bubble bath, get a haircut, or go for a walk in the park.
- Be positive and stay positive.
- Make sure you have a good set of scales for measuring all your foods.
- Make sure to weigh and measure yourself and fill in the sheets found in the back of the book.
- Make sure to make a note of you weight daily as well as weekly measurements using the charts at the back of this book. (See Appendix # 4 & 5)
- You may want to take some photos of how you look now and compare them to the end of the program. You will be amazed with the startling results.

- Shop in advance and make sure to have allowed food on the program readily available.
- Write a food diary; always be aware of what you are eating and the amount of calories being consumed as well as your fluid intake.
- Make sure you have prepared yourself a couple of days in advance to be properly prepared for every meal.

At the end of this book you will find a Weight Loss Tracking Chart, a Personal Measurement Chart as well as a Personal BMI calculator Chart. It is important to know your weight and height before you start this program and chart your BMI reading. You are to weigh yourself every morning once you have emptied your bladder. It should be the first thing you do in the morning upon rising and always wearing the same piece of clothing.

It is important also to measure yourself in order to truly see just how successful this diet is. Not only will you lose weight on the scales but you will also lose inches from your body. Simeons found that no matter how fat a person was, the greatest circumference, be it hips or abdomen, it will be reduced at a constant rate which is close to 1cm per kg of weight lost. For me this was certainly true. When I looked back over my before and after measurements I found that I had lost 20kg with a loss of 25cm from my waist!

SUMMARY OF ONE CYCLE OF THE PROGRAM

- DAY 1-2: Start taking hCG drops three times a day. Eat a normal diet with an emphasis on increasing fatty foods.
- Day 3-23: Begin VLCD of 500 calories eating only foods allocated. Continue hCG drops three times a day.
- Day 24-45: Maintenance Phase consisting of no sugars or carbohydrates, otherwise free to eat what you choose. hCG drops are no longer taken in this phase.

PART TWO

CHAPTER NINE

THE PROGRAM:
PHASE 1, STEP 1: LOADING PHASE

> **FIRST TWO DAYS ON OUR PROGRAM: LOADING PHASE**
> **DAY ONE AND DAY TWO**
> **YOU BEGIN TAKING THE HOMEOPATHIC hCG DROPS 3 TIMES A DAY**

In these first two days you are to eat as you normally do, with an emphasis on eating more fats. This is not the time to be counting any calories or starting a low calorie diet. Do remember you must start taking the drops in these first two days.

You must eat as much fatty foods as possible in the first two days of taking the drops. You are not to start the Very Low Calorie Diet (will always be referred to as VLCD) until day 3. It can take about two full days of taking hCG before the abnormal fat deposits are liberated and begin to circulate in order to become available as fuel for the body. By eating fats on the first two days you will not feel miserable and hungry on Day 3 (when you begin the VLCD) as the fat stores will be there for you. Simeons found that those that did not heed this advice were more irritable and less likely to adhere to the program than those that did heed the advice. He also found that those that did increase their fat content on the first two days, by day seven, had on average lost more weight than those that did not increase their fat content.

It is important here to increase the fats and not the sugars. It is also a good idea to increase good fats. One of the main reasons people are leptin resistant is due to the increasing amount of processed and chemically laden food. Use this time to start being healthy.

Eat more salads with homemade dressings (balsamic vinegar with cold pressed olive oil), avocado, nuts, olives; Omega 3 supplements (increase the dosage here for the first 2 days). Other fatty food recommended would be oily fish (and therefore not allowed in the VLCD when no fats are to be ingested) including anchovies, mackerel, salmon, sardines and trout. Try pancakes with maple syrup and butter or coffee with heavy cream!

Make sure to weigh yourself each morning and make a note in your personal weight loss tracking chart.

HOW TO TAKE THE DROPS

It is recommended holding the drops under your tongue for 10-15 seconds and then you swallow the residue. This allows the hCG to be absorbed directly into your bloodstream.

The homeopathic hCG drops should be taken at least three times a day. Some people in the first three to five days took the drops three to five times a day which helped to liberate more fat stores and therefore decreased hunger pangs.

In order for the homeopathic drops to be fully effective it is recommended not to take the drops with meals. If you are due to take some drops, for example at lunchtime, then take the drops 20 minutes before or after the meal. Avoid taking the drops after brushing your teeth if you use mint toothpaste or after tea or coffee.

PHASE 1, STEP 2: VLCD

> **BEGIN VERY LOW CALORIE DIET (VLCD).**
> **YOU CONTINUE TAKING THE HOMEOPATHIC hCG DROPS**
> **3 TIMES A DAY**

This phase lasts for 21 days and you keep taking the hCG drops three times a day. This is where you begin the Very Low Calorie Diet. 500 calories are to be eaten only and using only the foods listed (See appendix #1). You should refer to this appendix now to familiarise yourself with the foods on the program.

Your body shall receive very low calorie foods and a strict restriction on intake of sugars, starch and fried food items is imposed. You won't experience hunger pangs as the food reserves during the Loading Phase shall satisfy your hunger.

hCG breaks up and mobilises the fat deposits in your body and burns that fat for energy. 500 calories is giving your body its minimum food production allowance thus encouraging the body to burn the fat from your body for energy. Specific foods as listed cause chemical reactions in the body, combined with hCG to activate the hypothalamus, into releasing abnormal fat stores.

Although you may be concerned with your ability to survive on a VLCD (500 calories per day), remember that for every pound of fat that will be released from your body, it is equal to 3500 calories being released from your fat cells. Therefore your body is NOT functioning on only the 500 calories per day that you eat, but ALSO on the 1,500-4,000 calories per day that you are converting from your fat reserves giving the body much needed energy and nutrition.

In the Appendices (Appendix #2) is a calorie count sheet that you must refer to every day in order to ensure that you are eating at least 500 calories and no more than 550 calories.

Lunch and Dinner should each total around 250 calories. <u>Each</u> lunch <u>and</u> dinner consists of

- 3.5oz (100gm) of one type of protein food (A),
- One vegetable (B), and
- One fruit (D).
- The breadstick or Melba toast (C) are optional

The breadstick or Melba toast are optional but only one is allowed with each meal, not two eaten at one time. You must keep a record of what you are eating to ensure that you are not eating more than 550 calories or less than 500 calories.

Three egg whites must always be eaten with one full egg (totalling 4 egg whites and 1 yolk) to ensure you are getting your proper protein intake for the day. No more than one egg yolk may be eaten due to the fat content interfering with the success of the diet.

All visible fat must be carefully removed before cooking, and the meat must be weighed raw. It must be **boiled or grilled without any additional fat**. No oils are to be used in the cooking of foods. If you are able to access cottage cheese made from skimmed milk 100 grams may occasionally be used instead of the meat, but no other cheeses are allowed.

No ground (minced) meat or deli meats are allowed.

The juice of one lemon daily is allowed. Salt, pepper, sea salad vegetables, vinegar, mustard powder, garlic, sweet basil, parsley, thyme, marjoram, etcetera may be used for seasoning, but no oil, butter or dressing.

Tea, coffee, plain water, or plain sparkling mineral water are the only drinks allowed, but they may be taken in any quantity and at all times. The juice of one lemon (make sure to add the calories to your daily total) added to sparkling mineral water can be a fantastic treat in the evening. It is important to drink at least three litres of water a day in addition to any tea or coffee drunk.

The fruit or the breadstick may be eaten between meals instead of with lunch or dinner, but no more than four items listed for lunch and dinner may be eaten at one meal.

The two meals can be broken up. For instance having a breadstick and an apple for breakfast or before going to bed, provided they are deducted from the regular meals. The whole daily ration of two breadsticks or two fruits may not be eaten at the same time, nor can any item saved from the previous day be added on the following day.

Two small apples do not replace one large apple. There is no restriction on the size of one apple.

Chicken breast does not mean the breast of any other fowl such as turkey, nor does it mean a wing or drumstick.

It is important to remember that only **one** type of vegetable is allowed with **each** serving. You cannot have broccoli and tomato for example in one meal. You may on occasion, add 1 tablespoon of onion to a vegetable. If you need to make up calories, the best way is to make up soups and have them as an extra meal.

Only one tablespoon of milk is allowed per day. If you are used to milk in your tea or coffee it is highly recommended to have it black or switch to an herbal tea. A good idea is to save the milk portion for the day and have an omelette with the eggs. Keep in mind that if you do this, no milk can be used for anything else for the day.

Remember to write down your weight daily on your personal weight loss tracking chart and to measure yourself weekly filling in your personal measurement chart.

SAMPLE DIET DAY.

Breakfast:
Green Tea
Calories: Nil

Lunch:
One orange (69 calories)
100 gm Chicken breast (135 calories), 100 gm lettuce (20 calories)
Calories: 69 + 135 + 20 = **224** calories

Dinner:
One apple, large (110 calories)
100gm cod (95 calories)
Tomatoes (20 calories)
Calories: 110 + 95 + 20 = **225** calories

Additions throughout the day:
1 tbsp milk with coffee: 10 calories
1 fresh lemon juice with mineral water: 7 calories.
Calories: 10 + 7 = **17**

Total intake **224** + **225** + **17** (No bread sticks eaten) = **466,** therefore a deficit of **34** calories.

To make up the calories made up a broccoli soup of 90 gm (30.6 calories) with 1 tablespoon onions (5 calories), simmered in water and herbs. Soup was taken two hours after evening meal at 8pm.

Total calories = **35.6**

Total for day now: **467** + **35.6** = **501.6.** Perfect

ACTIVITIES TO INCORPORATE INTO THE PROGRAM

To ensure success on this program you need to incorporate the following into your everyday activities:

1. You must follow the program strictly without interruption for the first 23 days. This is the time when the hypothalamus and metabolism are improving, as well as leptin levels are returning to normal, unbound values.
2. Do not make any exceptions to the diet plan. Only eat the quantity allowed and foods that are listed in the program.
3. Success will depend on eating high fat foods on the first two days.
4. Success will also depend on following days 3-23 in Phase One as directed on the program.
5. Days 3-23 are when the hypothalamus is being repaired and reprogrammed. It takes this long for the effects on the hypothalamus to occur so it is very important to stay diligent with the program. The most successful and positive results will occur if you stay on the diet without any deviation on these days. It is during this time also that you will be reducing your food addictions to carbohydrates and fatty foods.
6. Purchase a food scale and make sure to weigh all foods raw.
7. No fat is to be ingested on days 3-23. If you are used to taking Omega supplements do not worry about stopping them while on the VLCD. The body will be able to survive without them for 21 days. Remember that while you are liberating fat stores you are also liberating stored Omegas 3, 6 and 9.
8. When you buy spices and herbs make sure that they have nothing added as some are sold with sugar added into them. Buy only from reputable health food shops as they are most likely to have only authentic ingredients without any hidden extras.
9. Make sure to do all your shopping from quality health stores, butchers, fishmongers, and green grocers purchasing organic produce as much as possible.

10. Remember, it is only for 21 days that you have to remain on the VLCD. Most of my clients stated that once they reached day five they were able to maintain the VLCD with the first couple of days being the hardest and did take some adjustment. In the first couple of days on the VLCD you may increase the hCG drops to five times a day. Twenty-one days is an attainable program, especially if it means a change which will be for the rest of your life. Do not give up. You can do it.
11. Women may continue to use birth control while on the hCG diet. Taking hCG will not affect the birth control. Even though there are currently no clinically proven side effects to our homeopathic drops, as with any diet, we recommend consulting with your doctor to make sure this diet is for you.
12. Mineral makeup is approved for use.
13. Most people continue to use their regular shampoo and conditioner while on the hCG diet. Avoid using any leave-in conditioners that stay on your scalp. Also make sure that you rinse off your conditioner from your scalp as much as you can.
14. Lotion should be avoided during the hCG diet. Do not use any body lotion while on the VLCD. Lotions contain a lot of fats and oils which can cause your body to retain the fats that you are trying to get rid of. A great alternative to lotion is organic Aloe Vera.
15. While on this program, intense exercise is not required. If you are already doing resistance training you will be building lean muscle mass which weighs more than fat with a differential affect when looking for weight loss. In the first week you may feel you do not have the energy to keep up with a vigorous exercise program. Pace yourself according to your own body's response. Do not introduce any new exercise regime in the early stages.
16. Make sure you are getting enough sleep. At least seven to eight hours a night is needed or else this can interfere with any weight loss recorded. You should find that while taking hCG that your sleep pattern will improve which also helps with decreasing leptin resistance.

17. Make sure you are drinking at least 2-3 litres of water a day. This is needed to flush out the broken down fat cells as well as assisting with energy levels.
18. Limit red meat to twice a week with emphasis on fish then chicken.
19. Consider taking supplements before the program to assist the body in making some necessary adjustments before starting the strict VLCD. See the Supplement Section (Appendix #3).

WHAT TO EXPECT ON THE PROGRAM?

Most people find for the first three to five days that they lose on average two pound a day with a large urinary output. After the fourth or fifth day of dieting the daily loss of weight begins to decrease to one pound or less per day, and there is a decreased urinary output. Men often continue to lose regularly at that rate, but women are more irregular in spite of faultless adherence to the program. There may be no drop at all for two or three days and then a sudden loss which re-establishes the normal average. These fluctuations are entirely due to variations in the retention and elimination of water, which are more marked in women than in men.

Some of my clients who had previously used diuretics, for whatever reason, lost fat during the first two or three weeks of treatment which showed in their measurements, but the scale may have showed little loss because they were replacing the normal water content of their body which may have been low. This is important to note if you were, or still are, taking diuretics for medical reasons. The lack of loss of weight on the scales should not be seen as a deterrent due to the fact that once your body is properly hydrated you will see a drop in weight on the scales. Fat is being lost but the body is being hydrated with water, which weighs more than fat. At this point you should focus in the loss of measurements in the body and how your clothes are fitting.

You may find yourself stalling and staying on the same weight for a couple of days. Do not worry. The weight registered by the scale is determined by two processes not necessarily synchronized under the influence of hCG. You may not be registering a loss on the scales but fat cells have been removed and you are in the process of relaying this on the scales. This is explained as follows. While fat is being extracted from the stored fatty tissue, these cells are being left empty. When they are left empty and therefore serving no purpose, the body breaks down the cellular structure and absorbs it. This is great news for you because this means that these fat cells cannot come back to haunt you in years to come by refilling. There is a fat extraction process going on here. The body needs to break up connective tissue and blood vessels which it washes out with water. Because water is heavier than fat, the scales you jump on in the morning may show no loss of weight even though the fat has been consumed by the body. When the tissue is finally broken down and the water liberated, there is a sudden flood of urine and a marked loss of weight.

Another reason for a plateau with weight loss is with women who may retain water just before their monthly cycle. Once their cycle starts, so too does a dramatic weight loss with the loss of fluids. So do not despair if you feel you are in a plateau with your weight loss while adhering to the protocol.

> ***Women lose an average 25lb in 23 days****
> ***Men lose an average 30lb in 23 days****

*Taking into account that everyone is different and these figures will only be achieved if program is strictly adhered to.

HOW TO OVERCOME ANY DELAYS IN WEIGHT LOSS WHILE ON THE VLCD.

Table 8: How to overcome stalling

TIPS ON HOW TO OVERCOME STALLING
• You may be unwittingly consuming chewing gum, throat pastilles, vitamin pills, cough syrups etcetera without realizing that the sugar or fats they contain may interfere with a regular loss of weight. Hence the need to stop taking these products. • Avoid starvation mode, and therefore no loss of weight, by consuming at least 500 calories a day. • Consuming red meat more than two times a week can slow down digestion. It is best to consume fish on a daily basis with chicken, red meat and eggs on alternating days. • On a daily basis, avoid using the same vegetable, protein or fruit more than once. • Use organic foods as much as possible. • Avoid using any canned products. All foods should be as fresh as possible. Canned goods have preservatives and flavour enhancers that may slow down weight loss as well as interfering with the repair of the hypothalamus. • Drinking herbal teas such as Yerba Mate, Pu Era, and Dandelion can help. • Try to exercise more, especially if you have not addressed a lack of exercise in your every day routine. Start out slowly with just small walks if you have never done any form of exercise. • Increase the green vegetables, except for cabbage which can cause some people to stall in weight loss. • Try omitting the breadstick or Melba toast. • Once or twice I cooked my chicken in coconut oil which was great in breaking a stall in weight loss. This should not be tried more than twice in a 23 day period.

> - If you have consumed all, or much of your abnormal fat then you may at once begin to feel much hungrier and even weak. It is important to be in tune with your body. For me, as I gradually came to within normal BMI, I had an increase in appetite but ignored the warning signs. I still maintained the VLCD, but was not losing any more weight. At this point in time, what I should have been doing was slightly increasing my intake in kilojoules. My body was registering that I had lost fat reserves and now it was time to hold onto some reserves. By increasing my calorie intake slightly, I overcame this obstacle. Keep in mind that this was at the end of my regime of three cycles and had lost a lot of weight.

Dr Simeons recommends doing an apple day if you have stalled in your weight loss. This would be indicated by no loss of weight in more than four days. He instructed his clients to eat six apples throughout the day (eating nothing else) and to decrease fluid intake to two litres a day. This works by assisting the body in getting rid of excess fluids that may have been the cause of stalling. As your system slows down on the VLCD, you may retain water. Apples have a unique ability of hydrating the body allowing you to shed the excess water. This should only be done maximum twice in a 23 day program and only as a last resort as you are only removing excess fluid and not fat cells.

CHAPTER TEN

FREQUENTLY ASKED QUESTIONS

WILL I BE HUNGRY ON THIS PROGRAM?

During the first week you may be hungry. Some people often refer it to an "empty feeling" rather than actual hunger pains. Those who ate more fats on the first two days generally complain less of hunger pains. Hunger is happening if the fat breakdown is stagnant. Increasing the dose of hCG drops to five times a day for a couple of days may help. Drinking green tea, Pur Erh tea or taking Green Tea capsules or Nopal capsules may assist. For further reference refer to Supplements: Appendix #3.

You will soon find the meal portions to be completely satisfying. This is partly due to your hypothalamus adjusting your metabolic rate, but largely due to the amount of calories circulating in your system from the fat being released. hCG opens up all of your fat cells. The liquid fat is then made accessible to the body to be used as energy. Even though you will be consuming fewer calories the body is able to access the stored energy that is in the fat cells. After a few days on The Slim Factor program, many of my clients reported a major decrease in their appetite, and plenty of energy to take on normal daily routines.

I AM SUFFERING FROM CONSTIPATION, WHAT CAN I DO?

Firstly it is important to remember that on a VLCD you will not need to do a daily bowel motion. Do not stress if you are going to the toilet only every two to three days, especially if you were used to going daily.

Supplements here to help would be Green supplements in capsules or powder form, Nopal, or Probiotics. For further reference refer to Supplements: Appendix #3.

It is important to choose your vegetables properly. Having greens every day would be ideal. Make sure if you are having green salad to include the bitter leaves such as endives and rocket.

Make sure to drink at least three litres of water a day. Adequate fluids promote adequate digestion and prevent constipation.

Exercise certainly helps to keep you regular while on the VLCD. Start in small stages if you did not exercise before starting this program, such as a walk around the block for ten minutes every day can be a great help.

WHY DO I HAVE MUSCLE FATIGUE?

Towards the end of the 23 day program you may find lifting things or climbing stairs require a great muscular effort. This is due to the removal of fat deposited between, in and around the muscles. According to Simeons, the removal of this fat makes the muscles too long and therefore have to perform greater contraction than before when performing a task. This issue will resolve itself in a couple of days as you go about your daily activities and exercise the muscles.

WHY AM I SUFFERING FROM HEADACHES?

Many people complain of headaches in the first couple of days. This is due to the body detoxing all the sugars and chemicals you have been feeding it in the past. If you understand that this is all part of the process then people can usually cope with it. Make sure to keep up your fluids to flush out all the toxins that are contributing to creating the headache. I am too much of a purist and will not take anything for a headache, but rather let nature take its course. For some people this is not an option and therefore should take whatever over-the-counter remedy they usually take for relief of headaches.

WILL I SUFFER WITH SAGGING SKIN ONCE THE WEIGHT IS LOST?

Keep in mind that it is not structural fat that is lost but the deep areas of stored fat. The normal fat stays intact and the skin usually shrinks with your weight loss, thus decreasing the appearance of cellulite. Body fat is properly redistributed and firmness is regained in the body.

SOME DIET PROTOCOLS PROMOTE THE USE OF STEVIA, WHY IS THIS NOT INCLUDED IN THE SLIM FACTOR PROGRAM?

Stevia is another chemical sugar. I do not care for all the research on it being zero calories and so on. A lot of modern day problems stem from the fact of using alternative sugars. You will notice that this program promotes only healthy foods. No additives are recommended. All foods are fresh, organic where possible, and unadulterated. Only meats, fruits and vegetables are eaten, no processed foods at all. It is in the processed foods that you will find MSG, additives, sweeteners, and so forth. My aim is to get you back to appreciating food as it should be. This means decreasing your reliance on sweet foods. Some programs promote Stevia in nearly every food eaten, thus creating a transfer of attachment from sugars to Stevia, not really addressing the need to remove our reliance on sugars.

A great natural sweetener is the spice cinnamon. Cinnamon can be added to apples for example if you are looking for a sweet treat. (See Recipes in Chapter #15)

CAN I DO THE PROGRAM IF I AM PREGNANT?

The short answer here is no. Your body is releasing toxins as well as fat stores. This is not the time to be thinking of you and losing weight. If you are planning on getting pregnant then do not start the program. If you want to lose weight in order to improve your chances of becoming pregnant, or want to lose weight before getting pregnant then make sure to use protection while on this program.

If you discover you are pregnant while on the program, stop taking your HCG and resume a normal diet.

WHY AM I EXPERIENCING LEG CRAMPS?

The most common mineral deficiencies that contribute to experiencing leg cramps are magnesium and potassium. With the large amounts of fluid being taken in and thus eliminated from the body, large amounts of minerals are also being eliminated especially magnesium and potassium. Some of my clients found they needed magnesium supplements while others maintained they avoided any leg cramps by supplementing with a good quality vitamin and mineral supplement.

Magnesium oil or flakes added to the bath, are a great way to relax in the evening as well as replenishing magnesium lost. Magnesium bath soaks are also recommended not only for the prevention of leg cramps but also to help you to relax if you are feeling stressed at any point in the program. My nightly pampering in the bath, with magnesium flakes added to the bath water, did much for my morale during the program.

As an alternative, magnesium oil sprayed on the body every evening helps. For more information on magnesium refer to Supplements: Appendix #3.

IF hCG IS RELEASED DURING PREGNANCY THEN WHY ARE PREGNANT WOMEN NOT LOSING WEIGHT DURING THEIR PREGNANCY?

This is the crux of the Slim Factor Program. hCG will only unlock the fat stores once the body's intake of food is limited to 500 calories per day. Fat tissue is only made available when calories are not otherwise available, as occurs when on a VLCD. If you tried to take the drops and not limit your calorie intake then the fat reserves would not be accessed due to the body getting enough caloric intake from the diet.

Most women, when they are pregnant, eat a normal diet so therefore are getting plenty of energy resources from their diet intake and do not need to draw from fat reserves, hence no dramatic loss in body weight due to circulating hCG .

WHAT DO I DO IF I WANT TO LOSE MORE WEIGHT?

If you want to lose more pounds and want to remain on The Slim Factor program, then you do not have to do the maintenance program at this stage. You may decide to take a break for a week from the VLCD, but may not introduce sugars or carbohydrates at this time.

You then repeat Phase 1 of The Slim Factor program. You should only do Phase One a maximum of three times to be strictly followed by the 21 day Maintenance Phase before returning to a normal eating program as explained in the Program For the Rest of Your Life in Chapter Twelve.

The reason behind the limit of three VLCD sessions is that this is long enough to be on a strict no carbohydrates no sugar plan. By all means, you may begin another program after a break of a couple of months if you have a more weight to lose. Keep in mind though, that after the maintenance program and with healthy eating and exercise you will be losing weight at a steady, albeit slower pace.

> **Once you have finished with Phase One, you are now ready to begin the Maintenance Program which is just as important.**
> **You are to stop taking the hCG drops after day 23.**

CHAPTER ELEVEN

PHASE 2: MAINTENANCE PHASE

> **YOU ARE TO STOP TAKING THE HOMEOPATHIC hCG DROPS**

For the past 21 days, you have been reshaping your body, nurturing your adrenal and thyroid glands, balancing your hormones (both male and female) resetting your appetite eating capacity, flushing dead fat cells from your system and most importantly losing pounds and inches.

The Maintenance Phase is responsible for stabilising your metabolism, targeting how your body is going to handle fats and carbohydrates from this point forward. Do not under estimate the importance of this stage. It is very crucial that it is adhered to, in order to ensure success of the whole program. If you do not do this phase correctly, you will be in danger of converting carbohydrates to fat, which is what caused you to be overweight in the first place. Sugar and starch are strictly restricted during the Maintenance Phase. Apart from that you are encourage to eat what you like, especially plenty of fresh fruit and vegetables.

> **CAUTION: STOP TAKING THE hCG DROPS FROM NOW ON.**

RESETTING YOUR SET POINT

The next phase of The Slim Factor program is the 21 day Maintenance Phase. This phase encourages long term good leptin behaviour which will protect you from rebound weight gain as well as resetting your new set point. Your new set point will be the weight your body now accepts as your normal weight as well as resetting your metabolism at a new, higher metabolic rate. It takes about 21 days for your weight to stabilize after the 21 day VLCD. The hypothalamus needs time to adjust to the new "set" weight if it is to be considered your "normal" weight. If you do not allow this three week period of maintaining the weight from day 23, it may be much easier to gain weight in the future.

On completion of this program the hypothalamus will be reset and corrected from its abnormal operating state. In the hypothalamus, leptin establishes the set point for weight limit. When it registers your set point at a certain level, it then dictates to the body how much fat should be in storage and how fast your metabolism should be. Increased metabolism, decreased hunger and decreased food cravings should all now be in progress. Your body should now no longer store fat in the previous abnormal secure fat reserves.

You may now eat anything you please, except sugar and starch. Food and drinks to avoid include potatoes, all breads, pastas, rice and other grains, grapes, bananas, all processed fruit juices, soft drinks and beer. A glass of wine is allowed. If your liver takes in too many carbohydrates during this stage, it will convert the excess into triglycerides and push them back into the blood stream and then stored in fat cells. You did not do all this hard work only to have elevated triglycerides and increased fat storage to occur. It is at this point that you want to maintain your newly acquired fat metabolism as opposed to carbohydrate metabolism.

You must, without fail, weigh yourself every morning as you get out of bed, having first emptied your bladder. Make sure your scales are on a flat, hard surface and not on soft carpet which will give you incorrect measurements.

It takes about three weeks before the weight reached at the end of the treatment becomes stable. During this period you must be aware that carbohydrates, namely sugar, rice, bread, potatoes, pastries and so on, are by far the most dangerous. If no carbohydrates whatsoever are eaten, fats can be indulged in somewhat more liberally and even small quantities of alcohol, such as a glass of wine with meals, does no harm, but as soon as fats and starch are combined things are very liable to get out of hand. This has to be observed very carefully during the first three weeks after Phase One is completed otherwise disappointments are almost sure to occur.

It is important to not try and lose more weight during this maintenance phase as it will almost certainly be achieved at the expense of your structural and essential fat, rather than the non-essential (abnormal fat), which you do NOT want to do.

Be sure to make sure that you are eating at least 1200 calories a day on the Maintenance Phase. Do not try and stick to the 500 calorie diet because this will only cause you to gain weight and undo all the good work you have done.

Table 9: One cycle of The Slim Factor Program

ONE CYCLE CONSISTS OF TWO PHASES:
<u>Phase One consists of two steps:</u> 2 high fat intake days (Loading Phase) 21 Very Low Calorie Diet (VLCD) days <u>Phase Two involves:</u> 21 Maintenance days

FOODS TO AVOID WHILE ON THE MAINTENANCE PHASE

Avoiding sugar means avoiding ANYTHING with sugar or sugar alternatives. Such foods include biscuits, cakes, sweets, soft drinks, corn syrup, processed food, energy drinks, fruit juice, honey, sweetened yoghurt, donuts, canned fruit, ice cream, processed breakfast cereals, fruit bars. The list can be endless. The best thing to keep in mind is that most processed food will have sugar added in the ingredients. To be sure of what you are eating it is important to get into the habit of reading food labels. Check to see if sugar is added into a product before you buy it. Nearly every product in a can or box contains sugar in one of its many names. Read the label on everything you introduce during the Maintenance Phase. Not only look for the word sugar but also alternative sweeteners in any form are forbidden such as xylitol, corn syrup, glucose syrup or aspartamine.

Avoiding starch means avoid cornstarch, white flour, wheat flour, any flour, pasta, any bread or bread product, breadsticks, bagels, crackers, tortillas, porridge, rice, polenta, peas, corn, lentils, pita bread, pretzels, corn chips, potato chips, potatoes, pancakes, muffins, nearly all root vegetables, any breading on fish or chicken, grains, cereals, granola, cereal bars, popcorn, biscuits, taco shells, croutons and rice cakes. (These are some examples only. If there is something not on the list that is a starch, then it is forbidden).

Meats to avoid include deli meats, bacon, prosciutto, sausage, and hotdogs.

The vegetables that should be avoided during the Maintenance Phase include the following dense starches: Jerusalem artichoke, squash, beans, corn, legumes, parsnips, peas, potatoes, sweet potatoes and yams.

It can still be difficult eating out as most restaurants and fast food places add sugar to nearly every product to enhance both flavour and shelf life. Do not eat processed cheese as it contains unnecessary sugars and starches.

You must ensure that you eat at least double the protein you were eating during the VLCD. You need to eat at least 100–125 grams of protein. That is not weight, but grams of pure protein. On the VLCD phase you averaged about 50gms, so at least double that so you won't be protein deficient.

WHAT YOU <u>**ARE ALLOWED**</u> TO EAT WHILE ON THREE WEEK MAINTENANCE PHASE.

- Eggs
- Meat, chicken and fish; grilled, fried or baked (make sure you do not eat any breaded products).
- Oily fish is now allowed.
- Cheese (although take it easy introducing it).
- Cream, yes enjoy good old fashioned cream.
- Nuts, again introducing slowly.
- Nut butters such as cashew nut butter and Brazil nut butter.
- Plain, live yoghurt adding your own fruit.

Some sample foods on this phase include:
- Steak cooked in coconut oil
- Avocados
- As much fresh fruit and vegetables (avoiding starch vegetables) as you wish.
- Fish can now be cooked in butter, wine and herbs.
- You may drink white wine on a few occasions.
- You can cook your eggs in butter and make omelettes with vegetables and a little cheese.
- Use olive oil or coconut oil in cooking.
- Avoid the so called bad fats such as breaded fish, nuggets, and fried foods and so on.
- Eat more dietary fat as it can be the key to maintenance. Overall, eat the good fats and your weight goes down, try to limit the good fats and your weight will go up. Many people make the mistake while dieting of completely eliminating fats. Although you were avoiding fats for the 21 day VLCD, you are to introduce fats into your diet now, making sure they are good fats. The good fats include salmon, sardines, fresh tuna (not canned tuna), herring, mackerel, anchovies, sesame seeds, sunflower seeds, pumpkin seeds, flaxseed oil/seeds, fish oils, avocado, hazelnuts, pecans, walnuts and almonds. (See Appendix 3: Supplements/EFA)

Many people find that the Maintenance Phase demonstrates a change in attitude toward food. For example, not opting for a second helping of food, but only eating what is on your plate. You may find that you are not as hungry as you remember being before you started The Slim Factor program. Instead, clients on this program stated that they eat only when they needed to eat, with less raiding of the cupboards that may have been a problem in the past. An amazing aspect of this program that many clients expressed was the ability to rid themselves of their emotional attachment to food both during the program and afterwards.

Be careful of introducing too many new foods at once. I always recommend people to introduce foods one at a time, so you can determine if a certain food causes a gain or loss. Some people have trouble with dairy or nuts. Start with lean protein, fruit and vegetables during the first few days. Then, gradually introduce foods like nuts and dairy one at a time, so that if you react negatively it is easily identified.

Be careful of all flavoured and/or fat free yogurts, which invariably contain sugar, regardless of soy or milk based. All yoghurts with fruit added will have sugars to assist with preserving the yoghurt and adding flavour. You can use organic, plain, live yogurt and then sweeten it with fruit such as raspberries, strawberries, blueberries with a dash of cinnamon added if needed.

Do not ever, from now on, resort to fat free or low fat products. This is one of the biggest lies we have been fed. If yoghurt, for example, is lower in fat than regular yoghurt, it has been adulterated in a way that creates havoc in our bodies. It might be less in fat but it will be higher in sugars, especially chemically altered sugars. We all need fats to survive. By adopting a low fat diet you are not eating any good fats and your body needs the good fats. You also need fat in your diet in order to absorb fat soluble vitamins (A, D, E and K) from your foods. More on good fats vs bad fats in my next book!

If you are having trouble stabilizing your weight, begin by reducing the fats a little such as cheese or oil, and increase protein and vegetables. Some people, especially women, seem to be sensitive to cheese and the sodium seems to increase water retention leading to nominal weight gain (though not fat gain).

Don't worry about weight fluctuations (within two pounds or close to it) too much. Many people have unstable weight for the first week to ten days after the transition from the VLCD to the Maintenance Phase. It is likely to stabilize for you in less than a week, so don't get upset by the minor swings during the Maintenance Phase. By the end of the Maintenance Program you should not be two pounds more or less than your weight on Day 23.

For those who are experiencing fluid fluctuations, you can combat it with drinking a lot of water (more than two litres), drinking dandelion leaf tea, taking Epsom salt baths, and watching your salt intake.

PART THREE

CHAPTER TWELVE

PROGRAM FOR THE REST OF YOUR LIFE

Weight loss on this protocol does **NOT** allow you to eat poorly without consequences once the Maintenance Phase is completed. Ice cream and a diet high in carbohydrates will make you fat, regardless of whether you lose weight on this protocol or any other kind of diet. In the hypothalamus, leptin establishes the Set Point for weight when it registers your set point at a certain level and then dictates to the body how much fat should be in storage and how fast your metabolism should be. You will maintain your new Set Point forever only when you adopt appropriate lifestyle changes that support healthy weight management. It is only logical. If you do things that made you fat in the first place, then those same things will make you fat again. Now is the time to make some important lifestyle changes, especially changes in your everyday diet.

You need to make sure that you do not revert to bad eating habits in the form of eating highly processed foods, tinned foods, sweet foods, fried foods or junk foods. Hopefully you will be in tune with your body and want to only eat natural foods, more fruit and vegetables and fewer sweets. It is the additives in foods that create a lot of problems so you need to pay attention to decreasing your reliance on processed foods. You should also decrease your portions of starchy foods. Limit the amount of potato and pasta in meals, incorporating more salads and vegetables into the meals.

You need to make sure you decrease the following from your diet from this point forward: white "starchy" carbohydrates foods such as breads, pastas, potatoes, rice, processed breakfast cereals and granola bars (something we associate as being healthy). You also need to pay attention to decreasing cakes, pastries, sweets, biscuits, chocolate, fried food, fast foods, canned foods, artificial sweeteners and soft drinks. Learn to identify foods with high amounts of MSG and HFCS. You may even want to go one extra step and avoid foods with herbicides, pesticides, flavour enhancers and colourings. This may take some major adjustments, and should be done one day at a time. If you do make the changes you will very much reap the benefits in the long term.

After you finish the three-week Maintenance Phase, be sure to add your carbohydrates into your diet slowly. Take note of what makes you gain weight. Start with healthy low glycemic carbohydrates like oat-flakes, wholegrain spelt pasta or brown rice and learn to decrease the portion size of your carbohydrates. Fill your meal plate up with more vegetables and salads rather than potato or bread. Add nuts and seeds to your porridge in the morning.

Keep up the good work of herbal teas, water or whatever else you introduced while on the program. Increase the good fats which are effective at decreasing the chances of leptin resistance reoccurring. Try some good quality dark chocolate for a treat.

You can now eat any foods you wish to. You may choose to keep weighing yourself daily to ascertain how your body responds to any new foods that you have not eaten in a while, to see how they affect your weight. You need to adjust your intake according to what you discover about your own unique response to foods.

If emotional issues are not properly addressed then success of long term weight loss could be jeopardised. It is important to address any emotional issues that you may have; if this is something that you feel would be of benefit.

Fat free on a label simply implies that there is less than half a gram of fat per serving. You are more likely to gain weight using fat free products due to the fact that fat induces satiety and makes you satisfied with what you have eaten. If there is a shortage of fat in your diet your appetite will be increased. Also, most commonly, when fat is removed from a product another form of refined carbohydrate is usually added to give the food texture and balance. Low fat diets seem to be very popular these days. Eating a low fat diet can leave you wanting to eat more. We all need fats in our diet. Good fats actually maintain healthy leptin levels and decrease the chances of developing leptin resistance. See Supplements: Appendix #3, for sources of good fats.

Always try and include a protein with every meal to assist in stabilising blood sugars. Some examples would be adding nuts to porridge or tahini paste to a fruit smoothie. Protein is more satisfying than carbohydrates or fats, and thus may be the new secret weapon in weight control. By including a little lean protein with each meal you will feel fuller for longer.

Protein takes longer for your body to digest so it satisfies you for longer. Plus, eating enough protein helps preserve muscle mass and encourages fat burning while keeping you feeling full. So be sure to include healthy protein sources, like yogurt, cheese, nuts, beans, or lean meat at meals and snacks.

Learn to take time out for yourself, take time to breathe properly; you may be shallow breathing without realizing it. Take time out during the day to take a few deep breaths and relax. Do not allow stress to build up. Stress can change your attitude to food causing you to break your new healthy lifestyle with you eating the wrong foods, which will ultimately make you feel worse and creating more stress on yourself. Try yoga, meditation or something simple like walking. Try and put yourself first sometimes. Get a massage. Research has shown that the act of touch does wonders for stress release. A massage will help to loosen out any tension in the muscles. If stress is an issue learn to manage your stress, take on challenges only if you feel able to. Learn to say NO to other people and YES to yourself.

Avoid stimulants such as tea and coffee, flavoured mineral drinks and chocolate; try and keep these things to a minimum. It is important not to feel deprived though so do keep everything in moderation.

You should find that after completing The Slim Factor program, not only is your body reshaped, but your eating behaviours and appetites will have changed. With your hypothalamus reset, your metabolism will also be different from when you started The Slim Factor program. Most clients find that they are now able to eat in moderation without feeling the need to overeat.

It is important to weigh yourself every week from now on. When you have finished the program, as much as ten pounds can be regained without any noticeable change in the fit of the clothes and can be a slow process over a couple of months. The reason for this is that after doing the program any newly acquired fat is at first evenly distributed and does not show the former preference for certain parts of the body.

TIPS FOR A HEALTHY DIGESTION.

Now that you have finished the program here are some tips for a healthy digestion.

- Take one step at a time.
- Avoid artificial sweeteners, packaged foods and hydrogenated fats.
- Avoid MSG, a flavour enhancer and preservative most commonly found in processed foods, tinned foods and typically in Chinese food. MSG is referred to as excitotoxin. It affects the hypothalamus and is chemically addictive, leading to obesity as well as depression.
- Avoid fast foods and take away foods. These foods are usually laden with hydrogenated fats, sugars and MSG. They are highly refined with very little fibre content.
- Buy fresh produce and learn to cook it. Always ask for cooking tips from your local butcher or local health food shop to ensure cooking tasty, nutritious meals.
- Use 100% organic foods where possible.
- 70-80% organic dark chocolate is great to nibble on.
- Use natural sweeteners such as cinnamon, organic honey, raw organic cane sugar or organic maple syrup. All in moderation though, just because they are natural sugar sources does not mean you can eat more.
- Choose lean beef (such as sirloin); white meat such as chicken and turkey; fish fillets (not crumbed), nuts, cottage cheese, eggs, or a small amount of nut butters such as cashew nut butter.
- Learn to do "foodless" treats. Instead of opting for a chocolate bar or a slice of cake, try a bubble bath, a foot massage, a walk in the park, or ring a friend for a surprise chat (one who is upbeat!).
- Frequent people who are positive about you trying to lose weight. Sometimes people like you to stay the way you are because you are their comfort zone. Be strong and be YOU.

- Keep an airtight container of nuts and seeds mix handy. Have the fridge stocked with fresh fruit and salads if you do feel like a snack in between meals.
- Do not rush eating your meals. Make sure you reserve time in order to enjoy eating in a relaxed manner.
- Eat at the dinner table and not in front of the television, and avoid any telephone calls while eating.
- Eat slowly and when you are full stop eating, do not over eat.
- Do not skip meals as this just tells the body that it is going into starvation mode and will slow down its metabolism. Best to eat regular meals with healthy snacks in between to keep your combustion engine going full steam ahead.
- Epsom salts or Himalayan salts in a bath help to eliminate toxins through the skin, putting less pressure on the digestive system. 250-500gm of the salts can be added to a warm bath. Take note that the action of the salts will increase your body temperature so you may feel warm in the bath. You may add an essential oil such as lavender which is very calming. Some people like to rinse off the salt in the shower afterwards, especially if you suffer from dry skin. Otherwise wrap up warm and allow the salts to further infuse into the body. Make sure to drink plenty of fluids, preferably water, after the bath.
- Remember the 80/20 rule. Be good 80% of the time to allow for some 20% divisional treats.
- Make sure your gut is getting plenty of pro-biotics. This may be in the form of plain, live yoghurt or by a good quality probiotic every day before breakfast. Avoid yoghurts with fruit added to them. Once a fruit has been added, sugar is also added to act as a preservative. Always choose plain, live yoghurt and then add your own fruit.
- Give up smoking if you are smoking. If you do not smoke then avoid taking up the habit!
- Do not drink water with your meals. This acts by diluting the digestive enzymes which interferes with the digestion of food, causing food not to be fully digested. One glass of wine is okay with the evening meal if you choose to drink wine with dinner.

- Look at the food you are cooking. Cook using fresh ingredients as much as possible.
- Buy vegetables and fruit that look fresh, not wilted or faded in colour.
- Eat until you are comfortably full and avoid the need to finish what is on the plate. This will only place a further burden on the stomach.
- Try and cook as much of your food from scratch as possible.
- Make sure you have plenty of fibre in your diet.
- Protein with every meal helps by you feeling satiated thus avoiding the raiding of the cupboard in the afternoons and evenings.
- Shop at local farmers markets which are great for fresh, local produce. You are helping both the local community as well as promoting a healthier YOU.

CHAPTER THIRTEEN
EXERCISE

ARE YOU GETTING ENOUGH EXERCISE?

It is one thing to watch what you eat, but you are also going to have to get out there and get in some exercise. There are many excuses for not being able to exercise. The only response here is that you have to get out there and improve your exercise tolerance levels. You will also start to feel better about yourself, and will have healthier glow that everyone will comment on.

Exercise increases the efficiency of glucose disposal and increases the sensitivity of your cells to insulin. This means less fat being converted to storage in your body. Exercise increases glucose metabolism and increases the sensitivity of the cells to insulin thus decreasing insulin resistance. It also assists in decreasing leptin resistance.

You may be suffering from arthritis without realising it. It can be insidious and starts with a few aching joints. Exercise improves joint mobility and muscle strength. Your joints will say thank you when you lose weight when they do not have to carry as much weight around, making life a little easier for them.

Exercise is essential for weight maintenance. You must exercise at least thirty minutes a day, three times a week to get your metabolism going.

Exercise may be exhausting for you at first. Choose an exercise that you enjoy as well as being able to do. Whether the restraints are children, weather or enjoyment, you need to find something that suits you or else you will not maintain any exercise program instigated. You need to establish routines, know what you are going to do for the week and make sure there are no excuses for you not to exercise. You have to put in the time here, no more excuses.

Extreme exercises can have the opposite benefits of regular exercise by elevating cortisol levels, everything we are trying to reverse. So do not go too overboard and wonder why the exercise routine is not working for you.

Do keep in mind that your body may be well out of shape. Your muscles may be soft, joints will be stiff, heart and lungs will not be used to such effort. You may feel slow and awkward but I can assure you this will get easier the more you exercise.

BENEFIT'S OF WALKING.

Walking is the best exercise if you have never exercised before and the benefits include:

- Stimulates the mind.
- Decreases stress levels. Hence the needs to make sure that you are not using your exercise routines to go over your day's problems. Need to keep the mind relaxed and clear in order to get maximum benefits of decreasing stress levels.
- Improves circulation, mobilizing fat stores leading to decreased body fat.
- Assists with cholesterol levels.
- Assists in decreasing blood pressure.
- Increases the efficiency of workings of leptin, glucose and insulin in the body.
- Can be done with the children.
- No outlay of a gym membership.
- Free and readily available.
- If you have a dog, walking is a great exercise for the dog who will love you for it.

TECHNIQUES TO REMEMBER WHILE WALKING

- While walking, keep your head up and remember to relax the shoulders.
- Most importantly remember to breathe. Your body needs more oxygen to keep up with the increase with your circulatory system needs.
- Invest in proper, well supporting running shoes and try and find soft surfaces to exercise on.
- Move arms as well as legs while walking. When the left foot is forward make sure to swing the right arm forward and vice versa.
- Breathe in and out using your abdominal muscles, they need to exercise too.
- Be quick with your step, you need to get up the heart rate but do not overdo it in the beginning.
- Concentrate on making the steps quick but comfortable.

MORE REASONS TO GET OUT WALKING (JUST IN CASE YOU ARE STILL NOT CONVINCED).

- Increase and maintain bone density and prevent osteoporosis.
- Improve mental acuity.
- Reduce and prevent the risk of various cancers (including colon, breast, uterine), stroke, diabetes, heart attack, heart disease and arthritis.
- Improves oxygenation to the lungs.
- Improve the overall quality of life.
- Become more agile and feel "lighter."
- Become happier and have a better outlook on life.
- Improve blood circulation and oxygen to vital organs in the body.
- Increase energy and endurance levels.
- Feel good about your body & improve self-esteem.
- Attain permanent weight management.
- Improve skin tone and colour.
- Smooth cellulite and improve skin texture.
- Help alleviate depression.
- Strengthen, repair and boost immune function.
- Regular physical exercise will help prevent or relieve many of the common discomforts of PMS and menopause.
- Weight bearing exercises, such as walking, stair climbing and jogging can help prevent osteoporosis.
- Lower blood pressure.
- Improve vision and hearing.
- Slow the aging process.
- Improve hair growth and shine.
- Improve the quality of sleep.
- Improves overall general health.

CHAPTER FOURTEEN

SPECIFIC REASONS **NOT** DO THIS PROGRAM

- If your BMI value is lower than 20. To calculate your BMI see Appendix #6.
- If you are pregnant or breast feeding.
- Due to the fact that you have to follow a very low calorie diet, along with a low fat diet (which prevents the normal emptying of the gallbladder) it can sometimes trigger a gallbladder attack in some individuals who are genetically pre-disposed to gallbladder disease.
- Small stones in the gall bladder may in some people, who have recently had typical colic, can cause more frequent colic while on this program.
- Those who suffer gout could find their symptoms aggravated, or those who did not realise that they had gout may suffer gout attacks while on the program.
- Wait for three months post heart attack.
- It is recommended that those with a history of heart disease or very high lipids to skip fat loading. The reason is that fatty meals can put an immediate strain on the heart. The risk of heart attack is higher after a fatty meal.
- During the VLCD do not introduce a new exercise regime. You should be able to do most exercises while on the program if you already had an exercise program prior to starting The Slim Factor program. Walking, swimming, yoga or Pilates are a good idea to introduce if you would like to do something while on the VLCD.
- If you have any concerns make sure to work closely with your local doctor.

CHAPTER FIFTEEN

RECIPES WHILE ON THE VLCD.

- All measurements are taken as the final product. For example, if the recipe states one cauliflower (500gm), you must weigh only the ingredients used in the recipe, not the whole cauliflower with leaves and core.
- All meats are weighed raw with all fats cut off.
- All herbs are dry unless stated.
- Meals with an asterisk* denote they can be frozen.
- You may adjust your meal sizes accordingly. For example, make the soups in batches of different sizes. You need to make sure to make a note on how many calories there are in each serving for future reference.
- All vegetables will have the amount clearly stated. For example if one tomato (100gm) is asked for then make sure your tomato weights 100gm. If it is small, you may need to use two small tomatoes, making sure to reach the 100gms requested.
- Make sure to pay attention to the meals with vegetables included in them. You are not to add another vegetable portion for that meal.

SOUPS/JUICES

CAULIFLOWER AND GINGER SOUP 138 calories
Makes 4 servings each 34.5 calories

- 1 onion, chopped
- 1 teaspoon coriander seeds
- ½" ginger, grated
- 1 cauliflower (500gm)
- 4 cups of water
- Juice of 1 lemon
- Salt and pepper to taste

Sauté the onion, in a small amount of water, for two minutes. Add the coriander seeds and ginger and simmer for another minute. Add the cauliflower and mix for one minute. Add water and bring to the boil. Simmer for ½ hour. Once cauliflower is soft, put into a blender and pulse to desired consistency. Add lemon juice at end. To be divided into four servings.

*MID AFTERNOON TOMATO JUICE 65 calories

- 2 large tomatoes (300gm)
- Juice of ½ lemon
- 1 teaspoon fresh coriander, chopped
- 1 garlic clove, chopped
- ¼ teaspoon cumin
- ¼ teaspoon Worcestershire sauce (no added sugar)
- 1/8 teaspoon celery seed
- Salt, pepper, Tabasco to taste

Combine all ingredients and puree until smooth. Serve once chilled or pour over ice cubes.

*TOMATO SOUP 120 calories
Makes 3 servings each 40 calories

- 6 tomatoes (600gm), chopped
- 1-2 cloves minced garlic
- 3 cups water
- 1 teaspoon basil
- Salt and pepper to taste

Mix together tomatoes with garlic, water, basil, salt and pepper. Bring to boil and simmer for 20 minutes. Blend in blender and drink. Make into three batches of 40 calories each.

LUNCH/DINNERS

*CREAM OF CHICKEN CASSEROLE 160 calories
Note this recipe gives your allowance for protein and vegetable for one meal.

- Chicken (raw weight 100gm), steamed until cooked
- 3 stalks celery
- 2 cups water
- 3 garlic cloves, chopped
- 1 tablespoon onion, chopped
- ½ teaspoon parsley
- ½ teaspoon basil
- Salt and pepper to taste

Combine all ingredients into a blender and pulse. Pour into a saucepan and bring slowly to a boil, then lower temperature to simmering slightly for 30 minutes. Serve or put into freezer once cooled.

*CHICKEN MARINARA 180 calories
Note this recipe gives your allowance for protein and vegetable for one meal.

- 100gm chicken
- 200gm tomato, chopped
- 1 cup water
- 3 cloves crushed garlic
- 1 tsp oregano
- 1 tsp basil
- ¼ tsp chilli powder

Sear chicken on both sides for 2 minutes. Mix all ingredients together, bring to boil and then simmer for 30 minutes. You may need to add more water if you find the dish is too dry before chicken is fully cooked. Need to stay by the stove and watch carefully while cooking this dish to prevent the dish from drying out.

*CHILE GRILLED CHICKEN 140 calories

- 100 gm chicken
- ½-1 teaspoon chilli powder
- 1 teaspoon apple cider vinegar
- 3 cloves garlic, chopped
- 1 teaspoon oregano
- ½ teaspoon ground cumin
- Salt and pepper to taste

In a zip lock bag mix together all ingredients apart from the chicken. Cover chicken in some salt and then add to bag. Make sure bag is sealed and shake to coat the chicken. Place in the refrigerator and marinate for at least one hour. Once ready to cook, place chicken under hot grill until cooked. Can be enjoyed both hot and cold, whatever you desire!

*GINGER CHICKEN 140 calories

- 100gm chicken
- 1 teaspoon cracked black pepper
- 3 cloves garlic, minced
- 1 teaspoon fresh ginger root, grated
- ½ teaspoon basil
- 1 cup water
- Juice of half a lemon

Sear the chicken on both sides until brown for a minute or two on each side. Then add rest of ingredients and simmer for 20-30 minutes. You may need to add more water if you find the dish is too dry before chicken is fully cooked. Need to stay by the stove and watch carefully while cooking this dish to prevent the dish from drying out.

*LEMON CHICKEN SUPREME 190 calories
Note this recipe gives your allowance for protein and vegetable for one meal.

- 100 gm chicken
- 1 cup spinach
- 2-3 cups water
- Juice of 1 lemon
- 1 teaspoon thyme
- Salt and pepper to taste

Chicken is to be cooked either by steaming or boiling. You may dice or shred the chicken. Then mix all ingredients together and simmer for 20 minutes. Serve hot.

*CHICKEN ZEST 215 calories
Note this recipe gives your allowance for protein and vegetable for one meal.

- 100gm chicken
- 4 tomatoes (400gm), chopped
- 3 cloves garlic, minced
- 1 teaspoon oregano
- 1 teaspoon basil
- 1 teaspoon thyme
- ¼ teaspoon chilli powder
- Cracked pepper and salt to taste.

Pre heat oven to 350ºF (180ºC)
Sear chicken on both sides in a heated frying pan for a minute each side until just brown.
In a casserole dish place half the tomatoes then add chicken on top of tomatoes and top with garlic.
In a small bowl, mix together rest of tomatoes with oregano, basil, and thyme and chilli powder. Once mixed thoroughly, place mixture onto the chicken. Top with cracked pepper and salt. Cover dish with lid or aluminium foil tightly. Bake in oven for 60 minutes.

*SEAFOOD MEDLEY 175 calories
Note this recipe gives your allowance for protein and vegetable for one meal.

- 100 gm white fish
- 3 tomatoes (300gm), chopped
- 2 cups water
- 3 cloves garlic, chopped
- 1 tablespoon onion, chopped
- 1 teaspoon parsley
- 1 Bay leaf
- ¼ teaspoon oregano
- ¼ teaspoon basil
- ¼ teaspoon rosemary
- 1/8 teaspoon fennel seeds
- Salt and pepper to taste

Place all ingredients, except fish, into a saucepan and bring to the boil. Reduce heat, cover and simmer for 30 minutes. Add fish and bring to boil. Reduce heat, cover and simmer for 10 minutes. You may add more tomatoes if you wish to increase your calorie content of this meal.

LEMON GINGER ASPARAGUS SURPRISE 29 CALORIES

- 100 gm asparagus, chopped, with woody ends discarded
- ½ cup water
- ½ teaspoon ginger root, grated
- 3 cloves garlic, chopped
- 1 tablespoon lemon juice
- Cracked black pepper

Mix all ingredients except lemon juice and pepper bring to boil and simmer for 5 minutes. Place into blender to desired consistency and add lemon juice and pepper. Enjoy.

DESSERTS

Yes you can enjoy desserts on this program. You may opt to simply eat the fruit raw which is great, but for some variety and treats I have included some of the following recipes.

*ORANGE ICY POLES 69 calories per orange used.

- 1 orange, juiced
- 250mls sparkling mineral water

Mix orange juice with mineral water. Can be presented as a juice with ice cubes or pour mixture into moulds for making ice treats at home. For me this mixture made three moulds which meant three treats in one summer's day!

APPLE SURPRISE 110 calories

- One apple, large, peeled and cut into chunks
- Water, 20-40 mls
- ½ teaspoon cinnamon powder

Place apples, water and cinnamon into a saucepan. Simmer for 10 minutes, stirring occasionally but making sure to watch mixture. Serve warm.
For an alternative, you may wait for mixture to cool and mix with some ice cubes and pulse in a blender (that is able to pulse ice) for 30 seconds and serve as a chilled dessert. Either way is tasty.

RECIPES FOR THE 21 DAY MAINTENANCE PROGRAM

During the Maintenance Phase you are allowed to introduce fat into your diet which does allow you some more exciting recipes. For me, my first meal was roast chicken. I really enjoyed that chicken! As a treat for successfully finishing the VLCD, I whipped up a little cream and put in on top of my morning coffee. That was a very rewarding coffee and I can still taste it on my tongue.

You will find that you can eat most of the family meals as long as you are cooking from scratch and not cooking readymade dinners. In all processed foods you will find sugar and starches so the best way to avoid making any mistakes during the Maintenance Phase is to simply eat as you were on the VLCD with some adjustments and larger servings.

During the Maintenance Phase you can adjust the above recipes with more fat and protein added. This can be done with cheese, nuts, cream, sour cream, anything but sugar and starch.

One delicious recipe, that no-one in the house would eat but me, is the following Chocolate Cases. I found that after the 23 (VLCD) days my taste buds were changed. They were no longer dampened by additives and flavourings that we do not realise we are eating every day. The following was my treat and I could eat one a day and not put on any weight and I found them delicious. They did melt very quickly in my hands and that is why I suggest you putting them into patty pans, or bun cases, so the body heat does not melt them. There are no additives or preservatives added to these treats to stop the melting process.

ABSOLUTE SUGAR FREE CHOCOLATE CASES.

- 2 tablespoons virgin coconut oil
- 3 tablespoons pure cocoa powder
- Ground cinnamon to taste
- Pinch of ground cloves
- 1 tablespoon desiccated coconut
- Mixture of coconut flakes, cashew nuts, and flaked almonds.
- Grated orange rind to taste.

Melt coconut oil over double boiler then add cocoa powder. You may prefer more or less cocoa powder to oil, depending on your preference. Add cinnamon, cloves, desiccated coconut and orange rind and stir well.

In the meantime, place nuts into patty pans (or bun cases). I put in two of each nut (almond and cashew) and two coconut flakes into each case. I then poured over the oil & cocoa mix. Place into fridge and chill for a couple of hours to set. Enjoy the treat.

PART FOUR

APPENDIX ONE

DAILY ALLOWANCE

THROUGHOUT THE DAY	Only one tablespoonful of milk allowed in 24 hours. Must drink at least 2-3 litres of water a day.
BREAKFAST	Tea or coffee in any quantity without sugar.
LUNCH	100 grams of veal, beef, chicken breast, fresh white fish, lobster, crab, shrimp or 3 egg whites with one egg. (A) One type of vegetable only to be chosen from the following: (B) • Spinach, • Beet-greens, • Green salad, • Tomatoes, • Celery, • Fennel, • Onions, • Red shes, • Cucumbers, • Asparagus, • Cabbage, • Cauliflower • Broccoli. One breadstick (grissino) or one Melba toast. (C) Optional. An apple or a handful of strawberries or one-half grapefruit or one orange.(D)
DINNER	The same four choices (A, B C & D) as lunch.

APPENDIX TWO

CALORIC COUNT

Red Meat 3.5 ounces/100 grams
- Steak = 160 calories
- Sirloin Tip Steak = 130 calories
- Round Steak = 166 calories
- Veal = 110 calories

Fowl 3.5 ounces /100 grams
- Chicken Breast = 135 calories

Seafood 3.5 ounces/100 grams
- Cod = 95 calories
- Crab Meat = 128 calories
- Flounder = 90 calories
- Haddock = 88 calories
- Halibut = 110 calories
- Lobster = 119 calories
- Red Snapper = 110 calories
- Shrimp = 110 calories
- Tilapia = 94 calories
- Lemon Sole =116 calories
- Monk Fish = 96 calories
- Whiting = 92 calories

Eggs
- Eggs = 3 egg whites <u>plus</u> one egg white with yolk = 125 calories

Vegetables 3.5 ounces/100 grams
- Asparagus = 20 cal
- Asparagus 1 spear = 3 cal
- Broccoli =34 calories
- Celery = 15 cal
- Celery stalk = 6 cal
- Cabbage = 24 calories
- Cauliflower = 22 calories
- Cucumber = 12 calories
- Fennel = 11 calories
- Lettuce all varieties = 20 calories
- Onions = 17 calories
- Onions 1tbsp = 5 calories
- Red Radishes = 12 calories
- Spinach cooked (1 cup) = 48 calories
- Spinach raw = 20 calories
- Tomato = 20 calories

Fruit
- Apples (s)=55 calories
- Apple (l)=110 calories
- Orange=69 calories
- Strawberries (6 large)=36 calories
- ½ Grapefruit=50 calories

Extras
- Grissini Bread stick = 20* calories
- Melba toast = 20*calories
- 1 tablespoon milk = 10 calories
- Lemon juice 1 tbsp = 7 calories

*Check for calorie content as brands may vary.

APPENDIX THREE

SUPPLEMENTS

The following supplements are recommended to improve metabolic efficiency, improve blood sugar levels, and improve alkalinity thus further enhancing fat burning potential as well as supporting optimum nutrition. All these supplements can be accessed from our website.
www.dargan.ie

1. COCONUT OIL

Always use high quality cold pressed virgin coconut oil. Coconut oil naturally contains medium chain triglycerides which are easier to digest than other fats due to the fact that they are handled by the liver directly and then used by the body immediately as an energy source. They are also the preferred choice in cooking as the oils are not denatured at high temperatures.

- Stimulates metabolism.
- Improves digestion.
- Helps release fat cells.
- Gently stimulates the thyroid.

2. RAW APPLE CIDER VINEGAR (ACV)

Your digestion may have been sluggish before you commenced this program. As the VLCD is great for reprogramming the hypothalamus, in order to prevent the body metabolism returning to its sluggish state, Raw Apple Cider Vinegar is a must to include in your daily program.

Always make sure you buy a cloudy ACV and not a clear liquid. The cloudy residue is referred to as "the mother" and this is where the active residues of the natural fermentation process occur. The "mother" is actually formed by the beneficial bacteria which creates vinegar.

- Stimulates metabolism.
- Cleanses internal organs.
- Powerful in helping to release stored fat cells.

3. PRO-BIOTICS

Most people do not have enough beneficial bacteria in their systems to deal with digestive tract related upsets. There are some common conditions associated with a lack of beneficial bacteria. If you have poor skin, diarrhoea and/or constipation, slow peristalsis (how long it takes your food to be digested and eliminated), flatulence, bad breath, body odour, lactose intolerance, or a low resistance to infections in general, your body is telling you that you need more beneficial bacteria. The best way is to supply your body with natural probiotic supplements from reputable health food shops or eating plain, live yoghurt.

- Improves natural flora in the body to stimulate metabolism.
- Improves digestion.
- Assists in cleansing.

4. GREEN TEA (*Camellia sinensis*)

Green tea polyphenols (EGCG) are a factor in maintaining healthy leptin as well as affecting other hormone levels associated with regulating appetite. Scientists in Chicago's Tang Centre for Herbal Medicine Research found that EGCG was successful in treating leptin resistance by working on hormonal systems that control appetite and body weight. They also increase fat oxidation, inhibit fat absorption and assist in glucose regulation.

Green tea has also been shown to increase noradrenalin levels. Noradrenalin, a chemical transmitter in the nervous system, plays a major role in the activation of brown fat tissue. Brown fat tissue is the only metabolically active fat found in the human body. Activation of brown fat by increased noradrenalin levels is significant in the fact that it burns calories from the white fat commonly found around people's waistline, hips and thighs.

Green tea has also shown to have a positive effect on intestinal dysbiosis by raising healthy gut bacteria while lowering pathogenic bacteria in the bowel thus supporting a healthy gut flora.

- Stimulates cleansing of cells.
- Increases metabolism.
- Helps regulate hunger.
- Inhibits fat absorption.
- Assist in glucose regulation.
- Assists in burning calories.

5. NOPAL CACTUS *(Opunita ficus-indica)*

Nopal cactus contains a unique profile of high soluble and insoluble fibres. The presence of these fibres assists in preventing the rapid absorption of simple carbohydrates (sugars) into the bloodstream while digesting a meal. This allows for lowering the Glycaemic Index allowing for a more stable blood sugar metabolism throughout the day. If you suffer sugar spikes and slumps due to abnormal blood sugar regulation, Nopal cactus can help in stabilizing blood sugar levels which can be helpful if taken two weeks before the VLCD so the body does not go into too drastic blood sugar maintenance, allowing for a gentle change in diet.

Nopal cactus helps to decrease LDL cholesterol and triglycerides levels. It also has anti-oxidant and anti-inflammatory constituents which assist in preventing the primary cause of heart disease, in the form of cardiovascular inflammation.

The insoluble dietary fibre (commonly referred to as roughage) absorbs both water and toxins and along with soluble fibre, allowing for regular bowel motions. For many people with problems in maintaining regular bowel motions, Nopal cactus can prove to be a gentler and better alternative to psyllium for those with a sensitivity or allergy to psyllium.

The dietary fibres and mucilage that are found in Nopal cactus control excess gastric acid production as well as protecting the gastro-intestinal mucous membranes. Studies have shown that Nopal cactus actually stimulates the healing of gastric ulcers by soothing and decreasing gastro-intestinal inflammation.

The prebiotics found in Nopal cactus help to improve normal gut flora levels. The fibre content in Nopal cactus promotes satiety when eaten before a meal which can be beneficial in the first couple of days of the VLCD. Nopal cactus also assists in the breaking down and excretion of fat. It also provides vegetable protein that helps the body draw fluids from the tissues thereby diminishing cellulite and fluid retention. Nopal cactus works well in conjunction with The Slim Factor program with fat excretion and elimination as well as addressing any fluid retention issues.

6. GREEN SUPPLEMENTS SUCH AS SPIRULINA, WHEATGRASS, AND CHLORELLA.

Wheat grass naturally supports the body's cleansing ability, spirulina helps to strengthen the body, and chlorella also cleanses, alkalises and protects the body. Together they are a great source of vitamins, minerals, amino acids, essential fatty acids and antioxidants.

Spirulina is a rich source of protein and has a low glycaemic index. It is a rich source of phenylalanine which can help to suppress the appetite and reduce cravings.

Green supplementation assist greatly in helping in decreasing cravings for sweet or carbohydrate foods as well as supporting healthy liver function. The increased peristaltic action assists in alleviating constipation and normalizes secretion of gastric acids. They help in decreasing any hyperacidity which may be occurring, especially from a diet full of processed foods and living a stressful life (and who isn't in this lovely modern day society). Greens help to decrease inflammation, improve acid/alkaline balance and supports detoxification pathways.

7. HIGH QUALITY VITAMIN AND MINERAL COMPLEX

A good multivitamin and mineral is very much needed to ensure a good foundation in your body. Simeon's stated that you would be releasing vitamins from your fat stores but the amounts would be dependent on your diet before you started this program. If your diet was low in good quality vitamin and minerals, such as a diet consisting of high processed foods, then you will most certainly need a good vitamin and mineral complex. A good quality, multivitamin and mineral complex should contain the following ingredients:

Vitamins B3 and B6 help to supply fuel to cells, which are then able to burn energy. Vitamin B6 together with zinc is necessary for the production of pancreatic enzymes which are needed in digesting your food.

B3 is important in stabilising blood sugar levels.

B5 is involved in energy production and helps to control fat metabolism.

Vitamin C is a great antioxidant and stress healer.

Chromium deficiency impairs the body's ability to use glucose to meet its energy needs and raises insulin requirements. If this is occurring in your body then it is harder to burn off your food as fuel and more may be stored as fat. Chromium also helps to control levels of fat and cholesterol in the blood as well as controlling any sugar cravings you may be experiencing.

Zinc is an important mineral in appetite control and a deficiency can cause a loss of taste and smell, creating a need for stronger tasting foods, such as crisps with plenty of MSG additives.

8. CINNAMON
- Helps regulate insulin and blood sugar levels.
- Assists in stimulating the hypothalamus into being reset in a normal state.
- Normalises appetite and helps release fat reserves.
- Improves gastric acid secretions.
- Is a great way to add flavour to foods by naturally sweetening them.

9. ESSENTIAL FATTY ACIDS (EFA's)

Essential Fatty Acids (EFAs) are necessary fats that humans cannot manufacture, and therefore must be obtained from the diet. The two main families of EFAs I am going to write about are Omega-3 and Omega-6.

EFA's are required by the body to support the cardiovascular, reproductive, immune and nervous systems. They are required in order to manufacture and repair cell membranes, enabling the cells to obtain optimum nutrition from your diet as well as expel harmful waste. EFA does also play a major role in immune function by regulating inflammation and encouraging the body to fight infection. When you increase your intake of essential fatty acids you will notice positive results in your skin, hair and nails. Your skin will be soft and smooth, hair and nails will be stronger.

Alpha Linolenic Acid (ALA) is the principal Omega-3 fatty acid. The following list is the best sources of ALA:

- Flaxseed oil (flaxseed oil has the highest linolenic content of any food).
- Flaxseeds, flaxseed meal.
- Hempseed oil, hempseeds.
- Walnuts.
- Pumpkin seeds.
- Brazil nuts.
- Sesame seeds.

- Avocados.
- Some dark leafy green vegetables (kale, spinach, etc.).
- Oily fish such as salmon, mackerel, sardines, anchovies.

Linoleic Acid (LA) is the primary Omega-6 fatty acid. The following list is the best sources of LA:

- Flaxseed oil, flaxseeds, flaxseed meal.
- Hempseed oil, hempseeds.
- Pumpkin seeds.
- Pine nuts.
- Pistachio nuts.
- Sunflower seeds.
- Olives.
- Borage oil.
- Evening primrose oil.
- Black currant seed oil.

10. MAGNESIUM

The levels of magnesium in our food today are lower than from our grandparent's, or even parent's, generation. Mineral deficiencies in people can be attributed to low levels in our foods due to longer shelf life of foods, greater food processing as well as the impact of intensive farming. Other reasons include high consumption of junk food and increased dairy consumption.

Magnesium is essential for enzyme production, energy production, and fatty acid formation. It plays a major role in relaxing the nerves, muscles and blood vessels making it an important mineral for cardiovascular health.

The body needs a continual supply of magnesium in our diet which it may not be achieving due to the conditions of modern day life as stated above. Presence of food additives, heavy metals or over consumption of alcohol can also contribute to low magnesium levels. Having low magnesium levels in the body can give you symptoms such as fatigue, high blood pressure, osteoporosis, cramping (including period pains), restless legs, insomnia, migraine, anxiety, as well as acute or chronic muscle pain. Craving chocolate can be another sign of magnesium deficiency.

You can get magnesium from your diet from organically-grown foods, including mineral-rich sea vegetables such as Dillisk or Kombu. Spinach, cashew nuts, pine nuts, Brazil nuts, black beans and quinoa, are all good sources of magnesium. Whole, unrefined grains are also good sources of magnesium. Refined, steam rolled grains, as opposed to stone ground grains, (another reason for shopping at your local health food shop) are generally low in magnesium. When white flour is refined and processed, the magnesium-rich germ and bran are removed. Bread made from whole grain wheat flour provides more magnesium than bread made from white refined flour.

For optimum magnesium levels, supplementation may be necessary. Common forms of supplemented magnesium, such as magnesium oxide and magnesium sulphate (Epsom salts) are badly assimilated and may not be properly utilized by the body. Magnesium citrate is better absorbed but can loosen stools in some people. If your digestive system is not functioning to its best capacity then you may not be absorbing enough of the magnesium from your supplements.

The best way to take a magnesium supplement in my opinion is as magnesium chloride, also known as transdermal magnesium or magnesium oil. Magnesium chloride, although referred to as an oil, is actually a supersaturated brine. The purest natural form comes from the ancient Zechstein seabed in northwest Europe.

Magnesium chloride delivers high levels of magnesium with optimal absorption directly into the skin tissue, entering the cells with immediate effect. By applying it directly to the skin it bypasses the liver and heads straight for your body cells. You simply spray it onto your body and rub it in. Beware of cuts and sensitive areas. If it irritates your skin, shower it off after 30 minutes. If you feel pain or tightness anywhere, spray it on the affected area and massage it in.

Try adding magnesium chloride to your bath for a relaxing soak which is beneficial if you have sensitive skin. If you are spraying magnesium onto sensitive skin, dilute it 50:50 with water until you get used to it as it can sting, even on unbroken skin.

Magnesium chloride is available in a spray form (for spraying on the body) as well as in a concentrated oil/flakes (to be used in a bath). As with all supplements, make sure to read the label and dosage accordingly.

11. YERBA MATE TEA(*Ilex paraguariensis*)

Yerba Mate can be drunk both hot and cold, to alleviate fatigue, suppress appetite, stimulate body and mind, and boost metabolism. It enhances bile flow and speeds intestinal transit time. It also suppresses your appetite, boosts your metabolism and helps you to achieve a leaner body making it a great adjunct to The Slim Factor program.

- Increases energy without nervousness.
- Decreases appetite.
- Stimulates release of fat cells.
- Helps to stabilize blood sugar, suppress appetite and increase caloric burn rate.

12. PU-ERH TEA

Is a type of green tea made from a large leaf variety of the tea plant *Camellia sinensis.*

Pu-erh tea helps the body to remove toxins, is anti-bacterial, is anti-aging, controls hormone balance, controls body weight and removes body fat, strengthens the immune system, and reduces inflammation. Pu-erh tea is a naturally refreshing drink and taken on its own has no calories, so it's the perfect drink to keep you looking good and feeling fit while on the VLCD program as well as for the rest of your life. It may help with the following:

- Enhances Qi and life force.
- Lower blood cholesterol levels.
- Help boost the flow of blood and help enhance circulation.
- Aid in the proper digestion of food.
- Help break down and reduce fat in the system.
- Helps remove toxins.
- Helps heal aches and pains.

APPENDIX FOUR

THE SLIM FACTOR PERSONAL WEIGHT LOSS TRACKING CHART.

Starting on Phase One Day One, fill in your weight first thing in the morning. Do this on rising, straight after passing water and before you drink anything. Continue your daily weigh-ins until the end of Phase One remembering to jot your weight down each day. Make sure to use a digital set of scales and make sure your scales are on a flat, hard surface and not on soft carpet which will give you incorrect measurements.

DAY	WEIGHT	DAY	WEIGHT	DAY	WEIGHT
1		8		16	
2		9		17	
VLCD	▓▓▓	10		18	
3		11		19	
4		12		20	
5		13		21	
6		14		22	
7		15		23	

APPENDIX FIVE

THE SLIM FACTOR PERSONAL MEASUREMENT TRACKING CHART.

Be sure to measure yourself before you start the program and on days 7, 14 and 21.

AREA	DAY 1	DAY 7	DAY 14	DAY 21	TOTAL LOST
WAIST					
HIP					
INNER THIGH					
BICEP					
BUST					

APPENDIX SIX

THE SLIM FACTOR PERSONAL BODY MASS INDEX (BMI) CALCULATOR

BMI is the best indicator of your present weight and your target weight. It identifies the percentage of body tissue that is actually fat.

Your BMI is the ratio of your height to your weight and is calculated as follows;

*Substitute you own weight and height measurements to get your BMI.
<u>Metric</u>: Weight = ***68** kg Height = ***165** cm (1.65 m)
Calculation: **68** ÷ (**1.65** x **1.65**) = 24.98 = Normal
<u>Imperial</u>: Weight = ***150** lbs *Height = 5'5" (**65**")
Calculation: [**150** ÷ (**65**x **65**)] x 703 = 24.96 = Normal

    Your BMI =

How to translate these calculations into figures that mean something for you turn to the following page.

BMI	WEIGHT STATUS
Below 18.5	Underweight
18.5-24.9	Normal
25.5-29.9	Overweight
30-39.9	Obese
Over 40	Dangerously obese

*For some people who have a lot of muscle there is the need to take care when accessing their BMI as high results may not necessarily mean they are obese.

Muscle mass needs to be taken into account if this is an issue.*

CONVERSIONS

This program first originated in 1950 when all measurements were Imperial. In writing this book I was aware of the fact of trying to be up to date with the metric system with which I was brought up with growing up in Australia. The problem with this was that the program rolls better with imperial measurements.

For all of you who have made the switch to metric, or were bought up on metric I apologise for taking you back in time. Here are some conversions for you:

1 lb = 0.45 kg
14lb = 1 stone
1kg = 2.2lb
1 cm = 0.4 inches
1 inch = 2.5cm
1 ft = 0.3 mt
1 cal = 4.2 kJ
100gm = 3.5oz
1oz = 28gm

lb = Pound
Kg = Kilograms
Cm = Centimetres
Ft = Foot
Mt = metres
Cal = calories
Kj = kilojoules
Gm = grams
Oz = ounces

APPENDIX EIGHT

MONOSODIUM GLUTAMATE (MSG)

The original ingredient that made the chemically additive MSG was Kombu, a heavy kelp which makes the base stock of Japanese broths. A professor Kikunae Ikeda was able to isolate a chemical with a molecular formula C5H9NO4, the same formula and property as glutamic acid. To stabilise the chemical, Professor Ikeda mixed it with ordinary salt and water to make monosodium glutamate (MSG), which he then patented. Once full scale production was underway, Professor Ikeda found a cheaper way of making MSG using fermented molasses or wheat. Nowadays scientists have made the new discovery that almost any protein can be broken down to produce MSG.

To understand MSG we have to ask what glutamic acid (glutamate) is.

Glutamic acid is an amino acid found in abundance in both plant and animal protein. The body is capable of producing its own glutamic acid, and is not dependent upon getting glutamic acid from ingested food and is therefore referred to as a non-essential amino acid.

Glutamate is glutamic acid to which a mineral ion (salt) has been attached. If the mineral ion is sodium, then glutamic acid becomes sodium glutamate.

What is MSG?

MSG is glutamic acid that has been chemically produced. When glutamic acid is chemically produced, it differs significantly from the glutamic acid found in the body. Glutamic acid found normally in the human body is referred to as L-glutamic acid. Glutamic acid that is chemically produced is made up of both L-glutamic acid and D-glutamic acid.

Protein, found in many foods, contains **bound** glutamic acid, along with 19 other amino acids. Eating and digesting proteins in food does not cause any adverse reactions.

The **free, unbound** monosodium glutamate is the chemically produced MSG found in many foods today and contributes to leptin resistance and obesity.

There is an absolute explosion of hydrolyzed proteins on the market such as whey protein, soy protein and pea protein. Take the example of pea protein. If a pea was eaten as a whole, you have eaten the pea with all its constituents in one mouthful each component working in synergy with each other. When you ingest pea protein, you are ingesting a protein that has been hydrolyzed indicating that processed free glutamic acid is present.

Protein powders that contain glutamic acid are invariably processed free glutamic acid. You may not always find glutamic acid on the labels of protein powders. The important message here is that proteins should be ingested in the way nature intended and that is only from real food sources such as meats, beans and dairy products.

Reactions after high doses of MSG, such as those people may complain of after a meal at a Chinese restaurant, include migraine headaches, upset stomach, diarrhoea, heart irregularities, asthma, and/or mood swings. Did you know that more than 40 different ingredients contain the chemical formula monosodium glutamate (processed **free** glutamic acid) that causes these reactions? Chemically produced MSG can be found in tinned soups, salad dressings, processed meats, bread, chewing gum, ice-cream, baby food and soft drinks. It is a cheap and simple additive that makes food taste better (referred to as the unami taste) and is used in frozen, chilled and dehydrated ready to eat meals and most highly processed foods. You also need to look out for MSG derivatives in low fat/no fat foods where natural flavour is lost due to the extraction of fat.

Sources of processed free glutamic acid (MSG).

Information provided (with permission) by the Truth in Labeling Campaign. www.truthinlabeling.org (Accessed November 2010)

The list on the following page of ingredients that contain processed free glutamic acid has been compiled over the last 20 years from consumers' reports of adverse reactions and information provided by manufacturers and food technologists.

Names of ingredients that always contain processed free glutamic acid:	Names of ingredients that often contain or produce processed free glutamic acid:	The following are ingredients suspected of containing or creating sufficient processed free glutamic acid to serve as MSG-reaction triggers in HIGHLY SENSITIVE people:
Glutamic acid (E 620) Glutamate (E 620) Monosodium glutamate (E 621) Mono-potassium glutamate (E 622) Calcium glutamate (E 623) Mono-ammonium glutamate (E 624) Magnesium glutamate (E 625) Natrium glutamate Yeast extract Anything "hydrolyzed" Any "hydrolyzed protein" Calcium caseinate Sodium caseinate Yeast food, Yeast nutrient Autolyzed yeast Gelatine Textured protein Vetsin Ajinomoto	Carrageenan (E 407) Bouillon and broth Stock Whey protein Whey protein concentrate Whey protein isolate Any "flavours" or "flavouring" Maltodextrin Citric acid (E 330) Anything "ultra-pasteurized" Barley malt Pectin (E 440) Protease Anything "enzyme modified" Anything containing "enzymes" Malt extract Soy sauce Soy sauce extract Soy protein, Soy protein concentrate Soy protein isolate Anything "protein fortified" Anything "fermented" Seasonings	Corn starch Corn syrup Modified food starch Lipolyzed butter fat Dextrose Rice syrup Brown rice syrup Milk powder Reduced fat milk (skim; 1%; 2%) Most things enhanced low fat or no fat Anything Enriched Anything Vitamin enriched

By food industry definition, all MSG is "naturally occurring." Natural doesn't necessarily mean safe. Natural only means that the ingredient **started** out in nature, like arsenic and hydrochloric acid.

MSG reactions have been reported from soaps, shampoos, hair conditioners, and cosmetics, where MSG is hidden in ingredients with names that include the words "hydrolyzed," "amino acids," and/or "protein." This could explain why people complain of itchy scalps without realizing it may be the MSG in the formulas creating the problems. Remove any formulas with these words and you have your answer to a clean, tidy scalp.

APPENDIX NINE

HIGH FRUCTOSE CORN SYRUP (HFCS)

When I first started out with looking for items with HFCS content I was bombarded with so many different foods and how many different ways sugar was being mentioned. The important thing to remember here is that we should be decreasing our reliance on sugars, no matter what their form is. Do not be deluded in thinking that by substituting your sugars for a "healthier" alternative is the answer. Sugar is sugar, and needs to be eaten in moderation.

High fructose corn syrup is hidden by food and beverage manufacturers under many names. Some of these names are: chicory, inulin, iso-glucose, glucose-fructose syrup, dahlia syrup, tapioca syrup, glucose syrup, corn syrup, crystalline fructose and fruit fructose. The Corn Refiners Association would like to change the names that appear on labels with the term "corn sugar".

The biggest HFCS culprits are soft drinks, fruit drinks, sports drinks, flavoured yogurts, frozen food, canned food, breads, breakfast cereals, cakes, biscuits, crackers, ice cream, children's vitamins, cough syrup, condiments like tomato sauce, jams, jellies, syrups, some meats, salad dressings, sauces and marinades, and snack foods and bars. The list is endless.

Sucrose, or table sugar is made up of about 50% fructose and 50% glucose, and high fructose corn syrup is usually about 55% fructose and 45% glucose. With a difference of only 5% where is the problems you might ask? In sucrose, the fructose is bound to glucose, but in high fructose corn syrup, there is much more free or unbound fructose. Probably the biggest reason that high-fructose corn syrup is such a problem is that it is absolutely everywhere in our food supply, even in foods that one would not expect such as in low fat yoghurt, resulting in us eating large quantities of HFCS. It is important to read labels carefully, or simply stay away from all processed food by only consuming food in its natural state to be 100% sure.

High-fructose corn syrup is available in three different formulations: HFCS-90, HFCS-55, and HFCS-42. HFCS-55, the type most commonly used in soft drinks, is 55% fructose and 45% glucose. HFCS-42, used most often in baked goods, is 42% fructose and 58% glucose. HFCS-90 is used almost exclusively to produce the other two types.

Agave nectar can range from 56-92% fructose, depending on the brand.

GLOSSARY

Adipose tissue: fat containing cells arranged in lobules.
Adrenal gland: glands located atop of the kidneys. Responsible for releasing stress hormones.
Amino acid: building blocks of protein
Aspartamine: artificial sweetener
Augmented: enhanced
Autonomic: ability to function without any external stimulus. Works completely alone.
Basal: lowest level
Beta-endorphin: Promoting feeling of well-being and increasing relaxation.
Blood brain barrier: A physiological mechanism that alters the permeability of brain capillaries, so that some substances, such as certain drugs, are prevented from entering brain tissue, while other substances are allowed to enter freely.
BMI: body mass index, a formula for determining obesity.
Calcium caseinate: is a protein extracted from the insoluble portion of milk and purified in a chemical process.
Candida: common yeast normally found in the mucous membranes of the mouth, intestinal tract and vagina of healthy people. Complications arise when the growth is more than what is considered normal, called Candida overgrowth.
Carbohydrate: an energy source for the body consisting of carbon, hydrogen and oxygen.
Cardiovascular disease: an abnormal condition with dysfunction of the heart and blood vessels.
Catalyse: increase rate of chemical reaction.
Cholesterol: an integral component of every cell of the body. High levels of low density lipoprotein (LDL) may be associated with cardiovascular disease, whereas high levels of high density lipoprotein (HDL) appear to lower ones risk for heart disease.
Corn syrup: a liquid derivative of corn starch.

CRP (C - reactive protein): a protein made by the liver in response to factors released by fat cells
Curable: able to restore health
Deficit: any deficiency from what is considered normal
Desensitize: render a person insensitive or less sensitive to something, thus not responding correctly.
Dextrose: better known as glucose
Diabetes: a disorder of carbohydrate, fat and protein metabolism primarily as a result of a deficiency or complete lack of insulin by the pancreas or due to the body's resistance to insulin.
Diencephalon: portion of the brain between the cerebrum and the mesencephalon.
Disaccharide: simple carbohydrate formed by two monosaccharides.
E621: number code for food additive MSG
Endocrine: pertaining to a process in which a group of cells secrete into the blood or lymph a substance, such as a hormone, that has a specific effect on the tissues in another part of the body.
Endocrinologist: one who studies the endocrine system.
Endocrine organ: include pituitary, thyroid and adrenal organs
Enzyme: a complex produced by cells that catalyses chemical reaction.
Free fatty acids: by-products of the metabolism of fat in adipose tissues. These acids are described as "free" because they can be transported in the bloodstream without the aid of any other carriers.
Fructose: a monosaccharide found in honey and fruits (levulose) and combines with glucose to form sucrose.
Ghrelin: a hormone produced mainly by cells of the stomach and pancreas that stimulates hunger. Ghrelin levels increase before meals and decrease after meals.
Glucose: simple sugar
Glutamic acid: a non-essential amino acid
Glycogen: a polysaccharide (many sugars) that is the major carbohydrate store in the body.
Gout: a disease of inborn error of uric acid metabolism with symptoms such as painful swelling of joints, especially the big toes.
hCG: Human chorionic gonadotropin
HFCS: High fructose corn syrup
Hibernate: a survival mechanism used to cope with periods of low temperature and reduced food supply.

High fructose corn syrup: isomerisation of glucose in corn syrup to fructose creating high fructose corn syrup, syrup with high fructose to sucrose content.

Homeopathy: a modality of medicine on the theory of "like cures like"

Hormone: a chemical substance produced in one part of the body that regulates the activity of an organ or group of cells in another part of the body.

Human chorionic gonadotropin: a glycoprotein secreted by placental cells.

Hydrogenated fats: hydrogen is added to oils (in a process called hydrogenation) to make them more solid, or 'spreadable'

Hyperglycaemia: a greater than normal amount of glucose in the blood.

Hypothalamus: a portion of the diencephalon of the brain.

Inflammation: protective response of body tissues to irritation or injury. Symptoms include redness, heat, swelling and pain.

Insulin: a hormone secreted by the beta cells of the pancreas. Insulin allows sugars from the blood to be transported into muscles cells and other tissues where it is able for them to be used by the body for energy.

Intrinsic: denoting a natural quality.

Isomerisation: the process by which one molecule is transformed into another molecule which has exactly the same atoms, but the atoms are rearranged

Kelp: common seaweed used in cooking.

Leptin: a hormone that has a central role in fat metabolism.

Leptin resistance: high sustained concentrations of leptin from the enlarged fat stores result in leptin desensitization (resistance). The pathway of leptin control in obese people is flawed at some point so the body doesn't adequately receive the satiety feeling subsequent to eating, thus forever have feelings of hunger despite eating large meals.

Lipogenesis: the production and accumulation of fat.

Lipolysis: the breakdown or destruction of fats.

Malto dextrose: polysaccharide used as a food additive

Maltose: the least common disaccharide in nature

Metabolic rate: the amount of energy liberated in the body in any given time.

Metabolize: breaking down of carbohydrates, proteins and fats into small molecules.

Monosodium glutamate: a food flavour enhancer.
MSG: Monosodium glutamate.
Musculoskeletal: pertaining to muscles and skeleton.
Naturopathy: a system of therapeutics including nutrition, Herbalism, homeopathy and flower remedies allowing the body to heal itself by natural processes.
Obesity: an abnormal increase on the number and/or size of fat cells leading to increased adipose tissue mass.
Omega oils: essential oils required by the body obtained only in the diet.
Osteoarthritis: a form of arthritis in which one or many joints undergo degenerative changes.
Pancreas: an endocrine gland that secretes various substances such as digestive enzymes, insulin, and glucagon.
Peptic ulcer: ulceration of the mucous membrane of the stomach or duodenum.
Pharmaceutical: any chemical substance intended for use in the medical diagnosis, cure, treatment, or prevention of disease.
Psoriasis: common skin disorder characterised by red patches on the skin with thick, dry scales.
Puberty: period of life where the ability to reproduce begins.
Satiety: feeling of being full after a meal.
Serotonin: normal levels in the blood produce feeling of well-being, amongst other things.
Serum: the thin, clear and sticky fluid part of the blood that remains after coagulation.
Set point: point at which the body maintains a certain weight.
Splenda: alternative sweetener
Stroke: an abnormal condition of the brain where lack of oxygen supply occurs to the brain due to damaged blood vessels of the brain.
Sucralose: artificial sweetener, branded as Splenda.
Sucrose: a disaccharide sugar from sugar cane, sugar beets and sorghum and made up of one molecule of glucose and one molecule of fructose.
Symptom: a subjective indication of a disease as perceived by the person. For example, person feels pain in an area, pain is the symptom expressed.
Textured protein: meat analogue made from defatted soya flour. Also known as TVP.
Thalamus: an area of the brain.

Thermogenesis: production of heat, especially by the cells of the body.
Thyroid: a vascular organ comprising part of the endocrine system, found at the front of the neck
Toxin: a poison
Transfats: hydrogenated fats
Triglyceride: a simple fat compound consisting of three molecules of fatty acid and glycerol. They are the principle lipids in the blood where they are circulated within lipoproteins such as HDL (high density lipoprotein) and LDL (low density lipoprotein).
Uric acid: a product of metabolism of protein that is present in the blood and excreted in the urine.
Varicose ulcer: ulcer of a dilated vein.
VLCD: Very Low Calorie Diet.

RESOURCES

All products listed in this book are available from www.dargan.ie

Julie runs two very busy clinics on a professional basis. She also is able for consultations via online access.

BIBLIOGRAPHY

1. A.T.W. Simeons, *Pounds and Inches: A new approach to obesity.* Rome. Arti grafiche Sealia, 1971.

2. April Wilkerson. Oklahoma City doctor touts benefits of HCG diet. *The Journal Record (Oklahoma City).* Jan 27, 2010. Accessed 14 November, 2010. http://findarticles.com/p/articles/mi_qn4182/is_20100127/ai_n48974364/

3. Artemis P Simopoulos. Essential fatty acids in health and chronic disease. *The American Journal of Clinical Nutrition.* From The Center for Genetics, Nutrition and Health, Washington, DC. Accessed 14 November, 2010. http://www.ajcn.org/cgi/content/full/70/3/560S.

4. D. Belluscio, Leonor Ripamonte, Marcelo Wolansky, *Utility of an Oral presentation of hCG for the Management of Obesity. A double-blind study.* The Oral hCG Research Clinic. http://hcgobesity.org/research/index.html.

5. E. Whitney, S. Rolfes, *Understanding Nutrition. 11th Edition.* California. Wadsworth 2008.

6. George A Bray, Samara Joy Nielsen and Barry M Popkin. Consumption of high-fructose corn syrup in beverages may play a role in the epidemic of obesity. *The American Journal of Clinical Nutrition.* Accessed 14 November, 2010. http://www.ajcn.org/cgi/content/full/79/4/537.

7. Jeffrey M. Friedman, M.D., Ph.D. Laboratory of Molecular Genetics. Accessed 14 November, 2010. http://www.rockefeller.edu/research/faculty/abstract.php?id=41.

8. Julieta L. Maymó, Antonio Pérez Pérez, Víctor Sánchez-Margalet, José L. Dueñas, Juan Carlos Calvo and Cecilia L. Varone. *Up-Regulation of Placental Leptin by Human Chorionic Gonadotropin.* The Endocrine Society, Endocrinology Vol. 150,(1); 304-313. Accessed 14 November, 2010. http://endo.endojournals.org/cgi/content/abstract/150/1/304.

9. Ka He, Liancheng Zhao, Martha L Daviglus, Alan R Dyer, Linda Van Horn, Daniel Garside, Liguang Zhu, Dongshuang Guo, Yangfeng Wu, Beifan Zhou, Jeremiah Stamler. Association of monosodium glutamate intake with overweight in Chinese adults: the INTERMAP Study. *Obesity (Silver Spring).* 2008 August; 16(8): 1875–1880. Accessed 19th November, 2010. http://www.ncbi.nlm.nih.gov/pmc/articles/PMC2610632/

10. Ke Chen, Fanghong Li, Ji Li, Hongbo Cai, Steven Strom, Alessandro Bisello, David E Kelley, Miriam Friedman-Einat, Gregory A Skibinski, Mark A McCrory, Alexander J Szalai & Allan Z Zhao. Induction of leptin resistance through direct interaction of C-reactive protein with leptin. *Nature Med* 12(4):425-32 (2006). Accessed 14 November, 2010. http://www.cmdrchina.org/UploadFile/201061916145161.pdf.

11. Monell Chemical Senses Center (2009, February 23). Fructose-sweetened Drinks Increase Nonfasting Triglycerides In Obese Adults. *Science Daily.* Accessed 19 November, 2010. http://www.sciencedaily.com /releases/2009/02/090212161819.htm

12. *Obesity and overweight.* World Health Organisation. September 2006 (311). Accessed 14 November, 2010. http://www.who.int/mediacentre/factsheets/fs311/en/index.html.

13. R. Sood, *Textbook of Medical Laboratory Technology.* 2005. Jaypee.

14. S. Shalitin, M. Phillip, Role of obesity and leptin in the pubertal process and pubertal growth- A review, *International*

Journal of Obesity Related Metabolic Disorders 27 (2003): 869-874.

15. Sources of processed free glutamic acid (MSG). (Last updated June, 2010). http://www.truthinlabeling.org/hiddensources.html.

16. W. L. Asher, Harold W. Harper, Effect of human chorionic gonadotrophin on weight loss, hunger, and feeling of well-being. American Journal of Clinical Nutrition, (26); 211-18, Accessed 14 November, 2010. http://www.ajcn.org/cgi/content/abstract/26/2/211.

17. William Banks, Alan Coon, Sandra Robinson, Asif Moinuddin, Jessica Shultz, Ryota Nakaoke, and John Morley. Triglycerides Induce Leptin Resistance at the Blood-Brain Barrier. Accessed 19th November 2010. http://diabetes.diabetesjournals.org/content/53/5/1253.full.pdf